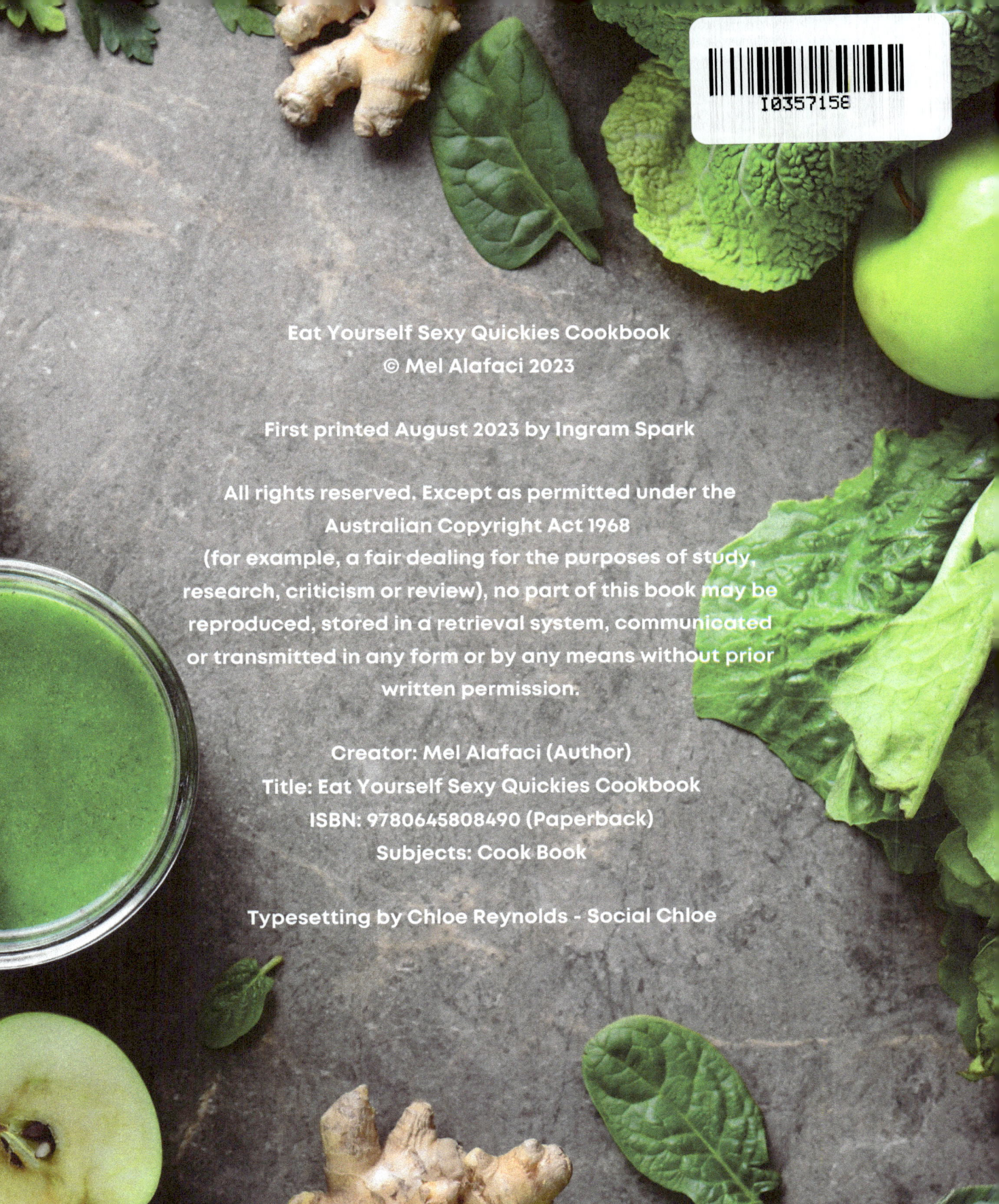

Eat Yourself Sexy Quickies Cookbook
© Mel Alafaci 2023

First printed August 2023 by Ingram Spark

All rights reserved. Except as permitted under the Australian Copyright Act 1968 (for example, a fair dealing for the purposes of study, research, criticism or review), no part of this book may be reproduced, stored in a retrieval system, communicated or transmitted in any form or by any means without prior written permission.

Creator: Mel Alafaci (Author)
Title: Eat Yourself Sexy Quickies Cookbook
ISBN: 9780645808490 (Paperback)
Subjects: Cook Book

Typesetting by Chloe Reynolds - Social Chloe

Chef Mel is taking on the WORLD!

With a smile that can light up a room, Chef Mel Alafaci has become a globally recognised chef and food educator. Her recent success in the USA means she's Australia's hottest rising culinary personality. Born in Zimbabwe, Chef Mel lived in South Africa before moving to Australia and starting her reign in the global foodie market.

She has an unwavering passion for cooking, eating, and teaching. And her intoxicating enthusiasm, authenticity, and unique culinary lingo will have you hungry to flex your muscles in the kitchen. Chef Mel is brilliant at adding humour, shortcuts, tricks, and hacks to all those tedious tasks, as well as making the scary ones simple and easy to accomplish.

CHEF MEL THE HAPPY CHEF | **@CHEFMEL_HAPPYCHEF** | **WWW.CHEFMEL.ME**

ABOUT MEL

Mel Alafaci has been passionate about food her whole life. She's the founder of Vanilla Zulu Cooking School, one of Australia's leading cooking schools, and has more than 28 years of professional cooking experience.

People battle to say her surname... so to make it easy she calls herself CHEF MEL.

WILD ABOUT FOOD!

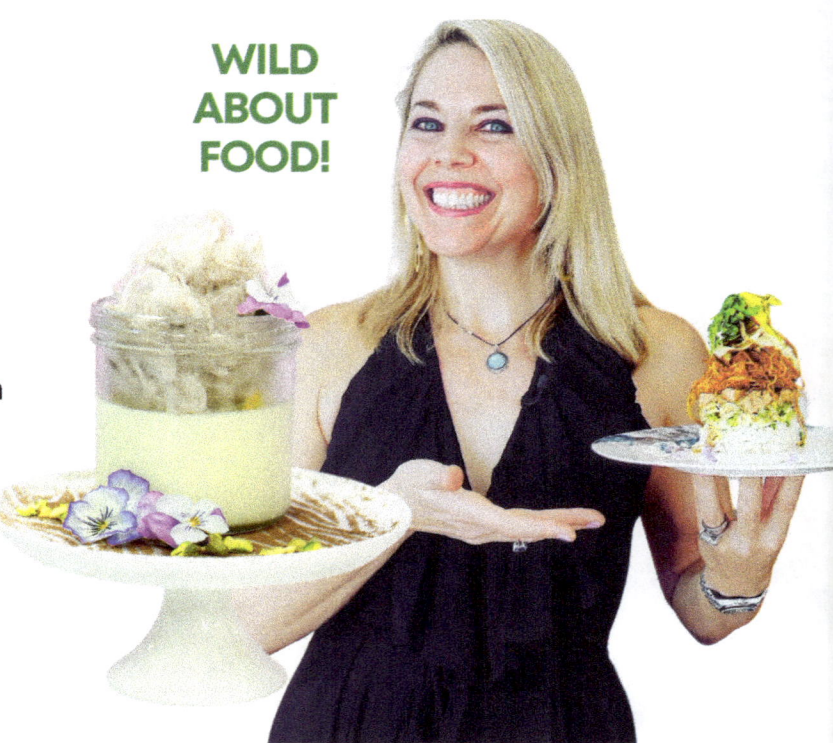

Before we begin..

1	Action Plan
4	Questionnaire
5	Mindset & Internal Language
6	Organise Your Wardrobe
7	Exercise
8	Your Fridge, Freezer & Pantry
9	Preparation Is Everything Eating
10	Schedule
11	Eating Out
12	Booze.. friend or foe?
13	Travelling
14	Snacking
15	Hydration
16	Shopping Lists
19	Eating Guide: Easy Mix & Match
22	Recipes

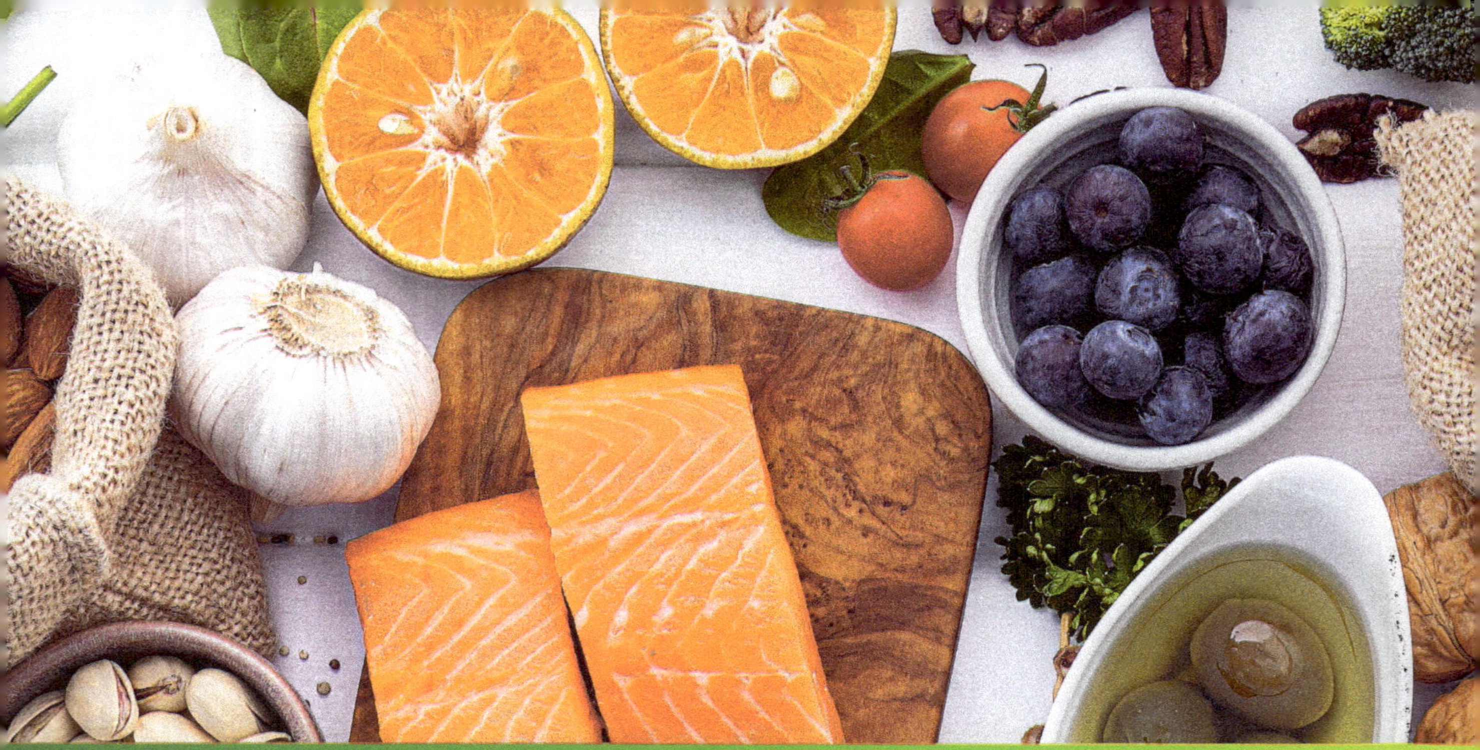

Action Plan

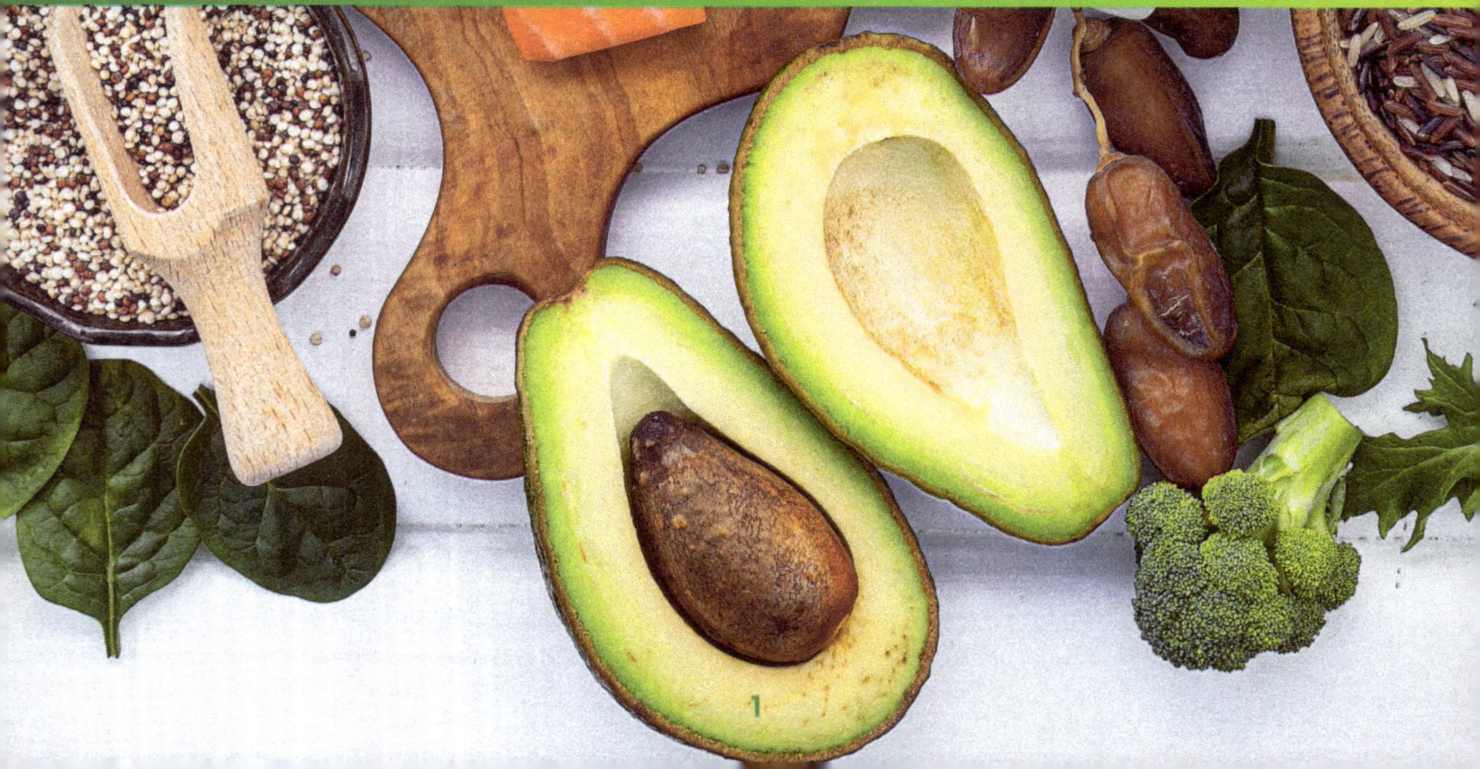

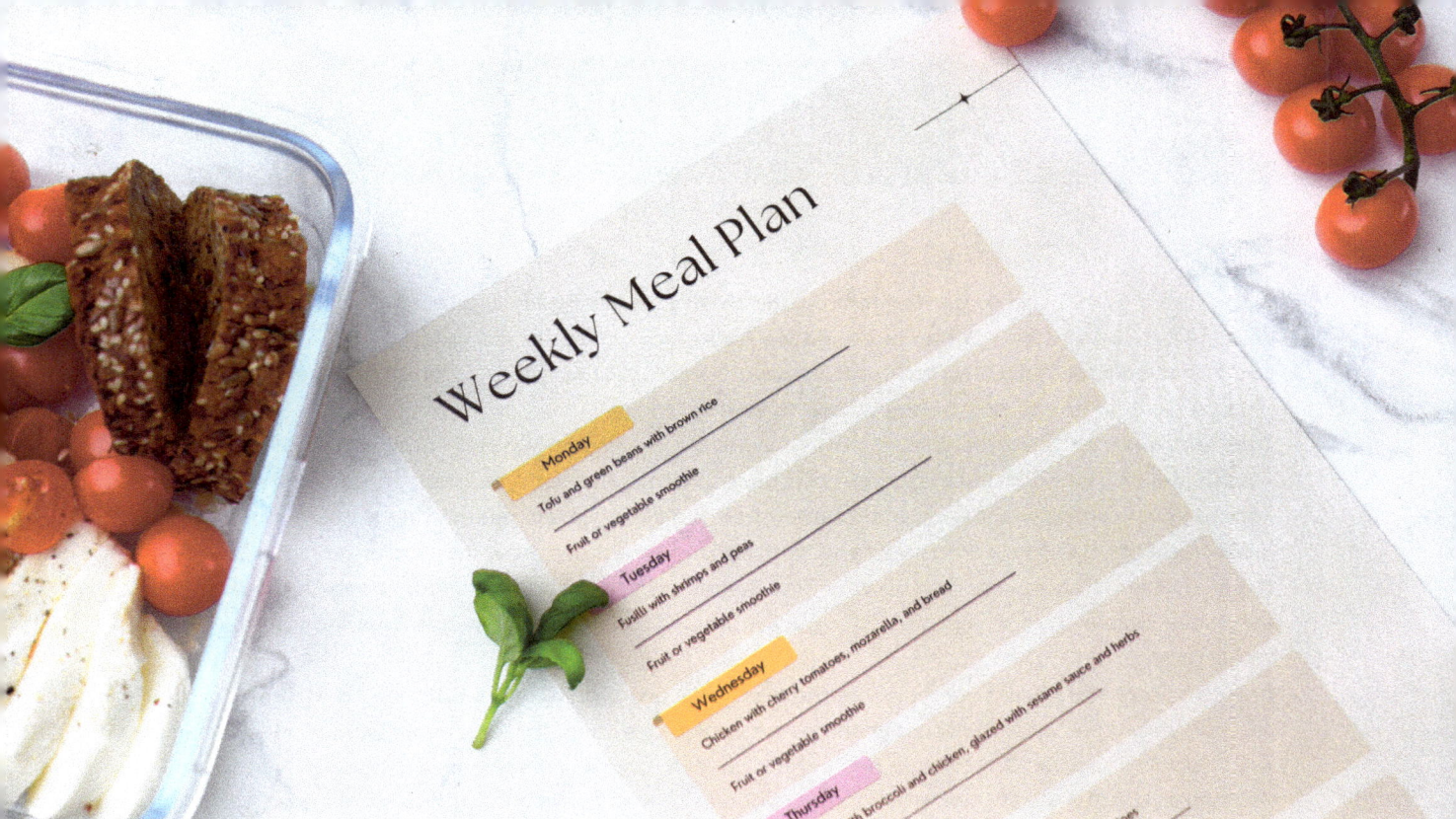

Every great success story begins with a great plan. Let's work on yours!

Here's your action plan for your 4-week Eat Yourself Sexy Challenge. After your kickstart, I encourage you to just keep going.

Once this new way of healthy eating becomes your normal everyday way, I recommend you keep going (with nice naughty cheat days thrown in once a week) so you really do live happily ever after.

Aiming for 6 days planned and healthy and 1 day off will make this so much easier.
It's important that food like cakes, chocolates, alcohol, and high-fat sugary items do become TREATS and that you avoid having them every single day. Remember, you are what you eat, and your beautiful body will only do what it's told.

It's time to do something for YOU. Time to cherish and value YOURSELF.

Give your body healthy, beautiful food and it will give you a healthy beautiful, sexy YOU! You deserve to feel good EVERY DAY. Mindful eating will change your life. When you actually MIND what you eat and are aware of eating for nutrition, success will follow.

Remember, before starting any new health or weight loss program, it's essential to consult with a healthcare professional to ensure it's appropriate for your individual needs and health condition.

Week 1

LET'S GET STARTED! YAY!
DISCLAIMER: PLEASE CONSULT YOUR GP BEFORE COMMENCING!

I'm so excited for you and thanks for joining my challenge.

- **Join the Eat Yourself Sexy Group on Facebook** For inspiration, support and fun.
- **Set Clear Goals for YOU using the questionnaire**: Determine your specific health and weight loss goals. Make sure they are realistic, achievable, and time-bound.
- **Take Measurements:** Don't panic, you are going to love seeing your weekly progress. And remember, if you have a BAD unplanned cheat day, you can re-commit and get right back on track the next day!
- **Record your starting weight, waist circumference, hip circumference and other relevant body measurements.** Use these measurements to track progress throughout the challenge.
- **Clean-Up Diet:** Start by cleaning up your diet. Remove processed foods, sugary beverages, and unhealthy snacks from your pantry. Stock up on whole foods like fruits, vegetables, lean proteins, and whole grains.
- **Create a Meal Plan:** Plan your meals for the first week, ensuring they are balanced and nutritious. This will help you make healthier choices and avoid impulsive eating. Try to get your whole family involved; it will be so much easier. Use the mix-and-match recipes I share in the Facebook group.
- **Go shopping:** Take the shopping list and get your healthy food into your fridge, pantry and freezer.
- **Do your weekly food prep:** Get chopping. Having healthy chopped and ready food is going to save you time and effort and encourage you to really get nutrition into your beautiful body. This is one of the most important and exciting changes you can make to your new Eat Yourself Sexy Lifestyle. Being prepared and having prep done WILL give you superpowers.

Week 2

START EXERCISING!

Begin with moderate-intensity exercises, like brisk walking, swimming, or cycling.
For at least 150 minutes per week.

Week 3

INTENSIFY THE EFFORT!

- **Increase Exercise:** Gradually increase the intensity and duration of your workouts. Incorporate strength training exercises to build lean muscle mass, which helps with fat burning.
- **Monitor Progress:** Check your weight, measurements and fitness improvements regularly. Use a journal or a mobile app to track your food intake and exercise routines.
- **Stay Hydrated:** Drink plenty of water throughout the day to support your metabolism and overall health.
- **Avoid** sugary drinks and excessive alcohol consumption.
- **Get Adequate Sleep**: Aim for 7-9 hours of quality sleep each night. Sufficient rest is crucial for weight loss and overall well-being.

Questionnaire

How do you feel RIGHT NOW?

It's essential to stop for a while and have a real heart-to-heart with yourself.
We have to see where we are to know where we want to be.

😊😐😞 MOOD
_____

😊😐😞 CURRENT WEIGHT
_____

😊😐😞 SKIN
_____

😊😐😞 HEALTH
_____

😊😐😞 FITNESS
_____

How would you like to feel on a daily basis?

_____
_____

What is your goal weight?

You have to have an idea before you start. Be realistic and don't be too hard on yourself.

_____
_____

What outfits have you stopped wearing because they don't make you feel good or just don't fit anymore?

Write down 3-5 items and get them back out...you WILL wear them again.

_____
_____
_____

Mindset & Internal Language

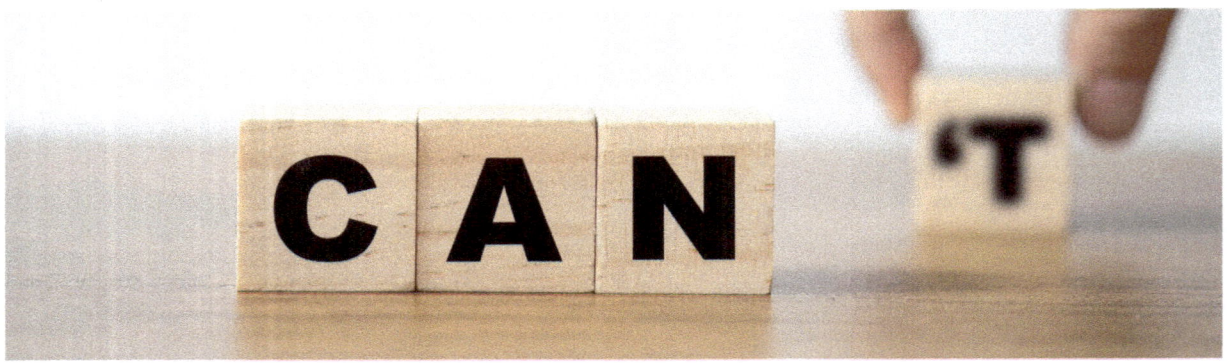

Guys and girls, you have to commit to prep.

If you fail to prepare, you prepare to fail. You HAVE to have your healthy options ready to go when hunger strikes!

Get your mindset right. You deserve this for yourself. If you are tired, lethargic or unmotivated, you need to do this. It's time to reward your body for being so amazing and so fabulous. It's time to get into that outfit you've been hiding in the cupboard because it doesn't fit you like it used to. Get your old self back...it doesn't take long to see AND FEEL results.

Remember, being sexy isn't about your weight or the shape of your body. Ultimately, it's how you feel about YOURSELF inside. That's what gives you that special glow, the one that everyone responds to. It's actually your happiness that makes you feel sexy inside and out.

I CAN'T STRESS THIS ENOUGH: If you fail to prepare, you prepare to fail. You HAVE to have your healthy options ready to go when hunger strikes!

We are also going to have **compulsory treats** as well as do some **fake drinking**. You don't have to stop drinking if it's all just too much, but you need to know that having a glass of wine or another alcoholic drink is like having a cupcake. We can't have too many of those or else it just adds up. Simple.
Retrain your brain.

Do this challenge with someone. It's always easier having someone to report to, or to discuss successes and failures with. I'll be here for you too...I'm only a DM away. (I seriously answer everyone...I actually care. Ask anyone.). You have to set yourself a realistic goal. It doesn't have to be on the scales...it can be that pair of jeans, that dress, that suit...I KNOW you have an outfit you've been keeping for years.

Try it on; it might not fit NOW but it will fit SOON. Every little step counts. Every little morsel you put into your mouth counts. Mindful eating. Mindful drinking. Don't think it doesn't count...it DOES.

Organise Your Wardrobe

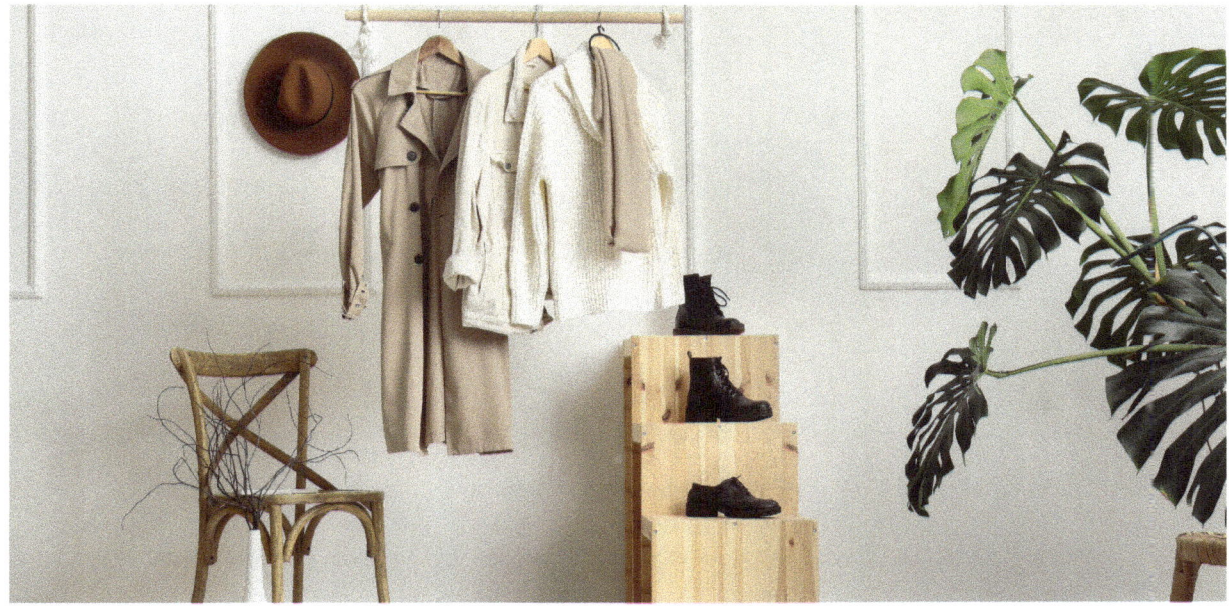

Listen up. This is about to get fun. I promise.

This might be an overwhelming task but you owe it to yourself. You owe it to the new you, the future you and I promise you will feel SO amazing afterwards.

It doesn't matter what time of the year you do this, but clean out your wardrobe. Take everything out and give it a good tidy. This will help you feel in control AND while you are in there I want you to set aside three to five outfits that you have stopped wearing and that you have been hiding at the back of the wardrobe or in a drawer because you can't face that they don't fit anymore. But do you know what that means?

It's good news. It means that somewhere deep inside you KNEW that you would claim yourself back. You KNEW that you were one day going to get yourself into the right frame of mind to succeed with your goals.

So get those outfits out. Try them on. Even if they don't fit, try them on. Take a photo. Every two weeks on your Eat Yourself Sexy journey you will try them on again and guess what? One sweet day, that suit or that dress or that pair of jeans will be back on that gorgeous body of yours. Having these garments in full view will give you the motivation and the courage you need to get you through the hard times. And there will be hard times.

When hard times hit be prepared, don't give up. Hopefully, by now you have joined the EAT YOURSELF SEXY group on Facebook...if not do it now. We are all here waiting to support you every step of the way.

Exercise

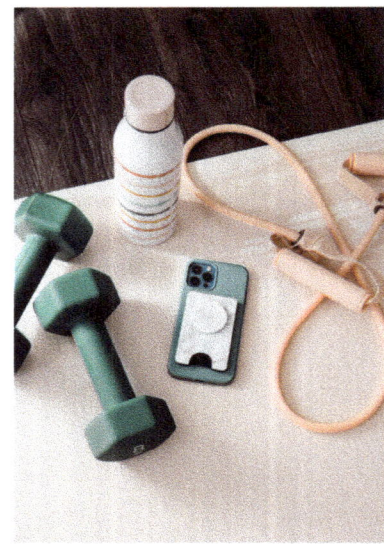 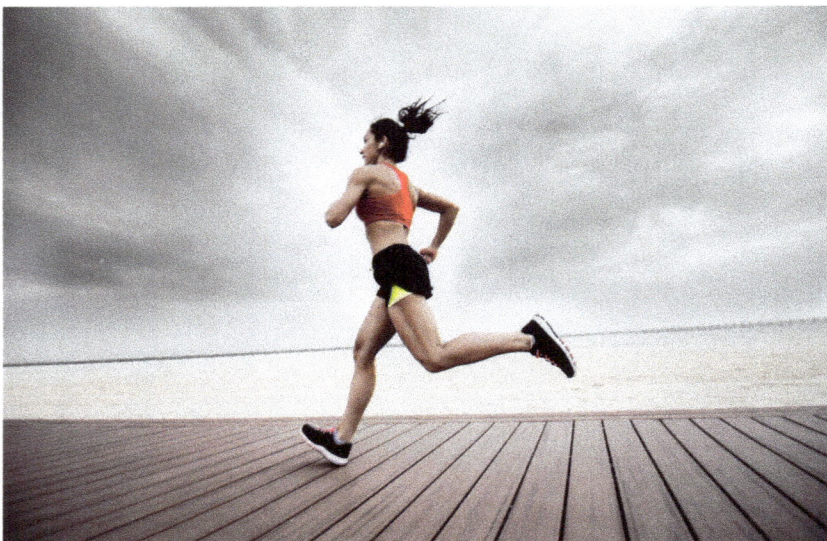

You cannot train off a bad diet.

You literally ARE what you EAT. Sexy is not only how you look, it's how you feel INSIDE.

You need to exercise. It's good for you. It's also the BEST thing you can possibly do if you are feeling down, stressed, angry or fed up. It can be anything your little heart desires.

It can be absolutely free or you can pay someone to train you and hold you accountable. That all depends on who YOU are as an individual. I personally need to pay someone to watch me and make sure I'm not slacking off. As a people pleaser, I feel ever so bad if I don't put in my best effort for my coach. I love to train with friends, I am just no good on my own, but many of you are. Do YOU! If you can afford to buy booze and chocolate, you can afford to join a gym or some form of fitness.

You can take the dog for a walk, start a couch to 5 K challenge, or sign up for yoga, Pilates, CrossFit or dance classes. Not only is this going to be good for your body, but 'workout time' can become your 'me' time.

Nothing takes the heat out of a work issue, a family drama, a traffic incident or daily stress like a seriously good sweaty workout. It really helps get rid of all that negative energy.

So even if you don't feel like it...get moving! You DESERVE some exercise, it should be YOUR treat, YOUR special time.

I train at least four times a week, it keeps me sane. I'm so much nicer to be around after a workout. Keep pitching up, you'll be surprised what a difference consistency makes.
Spend that money on yourself or do something free; 'something' is better than 'nothing'. COMMIT to your happiness now...I DARE YOU!

Your Fridge, Freezer & Pantry

Nothing, and I mean NOTHING, says 'I mean business' like sorting out your fridge, freezer and pantry. These are literally YOUR supply chain buddies to get as much healthy food in front of your happy face as possible. It's time to start using these to their fullest capabilities. It's time to feel fresh and in control.

Pantry

Spring clean your pantry, and pay particular attention to things that have expired. Sniff your nuts and your spices... stale pine nuts or a cinnamon from 1996 that you have kept for the last six moves will not be sexy anymore. Regift your old spices or throw them in the bin. YOU deserve better. Also make sure all your oils, tins and everything else is in date, and make sure you know what you have in those long-forgotten drawers and cupboards.

Fridge

I have a fresh take on how to arrange the fridge and boy does it differ from the manufacturer's vision. It differs a LOT. Don't worry about doing this if you don't have the same problem I had. Over the years I have realised that to me (and again this might NOT be the same for you) those crisper trays and veggie drawers are where my fruit and veg go to die. It's because I can't see them. They aren't in my face when I open those doors and the lights go on. The number of times I have gone to the fridge only to discover that my lettuce is limp, or that I've bought two more salad packs and have forgotten that there were three already there and now they are slimy and I've wasted all that fresh produce got too depressing and annoying. And yet, there the mustards and the pickles were with PRIME spots and how often did I use those? Almost never.

So here's how I have done it. I took everything out, cleaned it all and started with a clean slate. I put the don't-use-often things like the jars, the jams the tubes and the condiments in the drawers and the trays. I put the eggs and the cheeses and those more-than-a-few-days shelf-life things in the trays and the drawers too. I also keep my flour, baking powder and nuts in the trays...I live in a hot, humid climate and my packets of rice, pasta, flour and nuts do not last for months and months on the pantry shelf, so I gave those a new home in my sparkly clean fridge. By doing this I have literally saved myself a fortune and am no longer swearing profusely and cursing those damn weevils and moths.

The top shelf is the coldest, so I put my yogurt, cream cheeses, cottage cheese, fresh chicken or salmon or ham or mince, whatever I have out for the next few days to cook up. The next few shelves are adorned with my veggies. They are the FIRST thing I see when I open that fridge...it's like my conscience and also I can tell what needs to be used first because if I have done my prep and chopped veggies for the next few days, I can see what needs to be used first.

Freezer

I have the freezer in the kitchen allocated to things like frozen veggies, bulk nuts, bulk spices, bulk flour, frozen meat, and frozen ready-made meals from previous prep. It's essential to have frozen meals ready for the nights you don't want to cook. Putting your nuts and flour and spices in the freezer will extend the shelf life dramatically and save you lots of money.

Preparation Is Everything

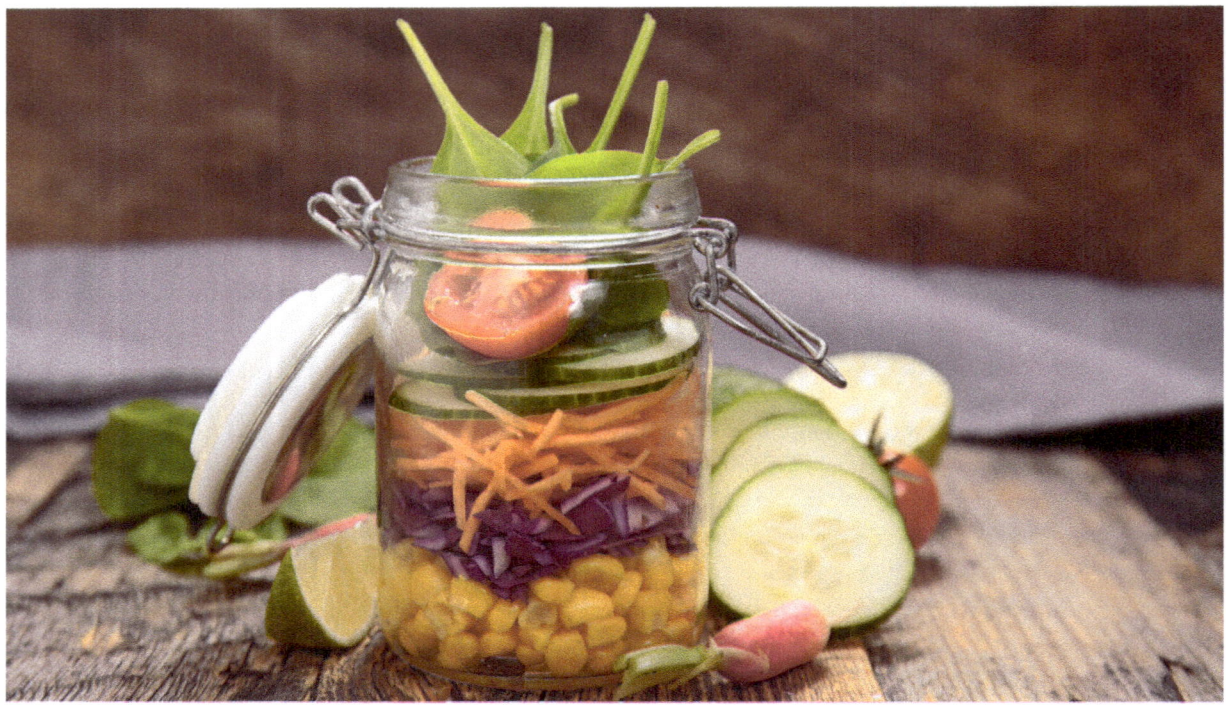

Set aside some time to do some prep.

We are going to chop and prepare some healthy choices so that when you're too busy, too tired or running late, you can reach for a planned healthy option. You owe it to yourself to put some effort in. If you're not good at chopping and it stresses you out, use your food processor or do yourself a favour and sign up for my free knife skills course. It's time you learned how to handle a knife. It's time you learn how to be efficient. It's time you learn how to be happy.

Once those salad packs have been used up in your first few days of the Eat Yourself Sexy Challenge, it will be time to chop up the head of broccoli, the cabbage, the carrots, and the capsicums/peppers. So, invest in some good airtight containers in various sizes. These will then be stored in your fridge in prime position so they are the FIRST thing you see when you open your fridge.

Keep your chopped veg separate or together depending on your personal preference, but make sure you do it. You can't eat yourself sexy if you don't have a healthy stash in the fridge.
Pop some salad and veggies in layers in a jar and top with protein. Perfect to take to work or leave in the fridge for when it's time to nourish!

NOW LET'S GET CHOPPING!
Don't forget to sign up for my FREE knife skills course. Head to my Instagram Bio, click the link, scroll down and sign up for the free knife skills course. You will be so happy you did.

Eating Schedule

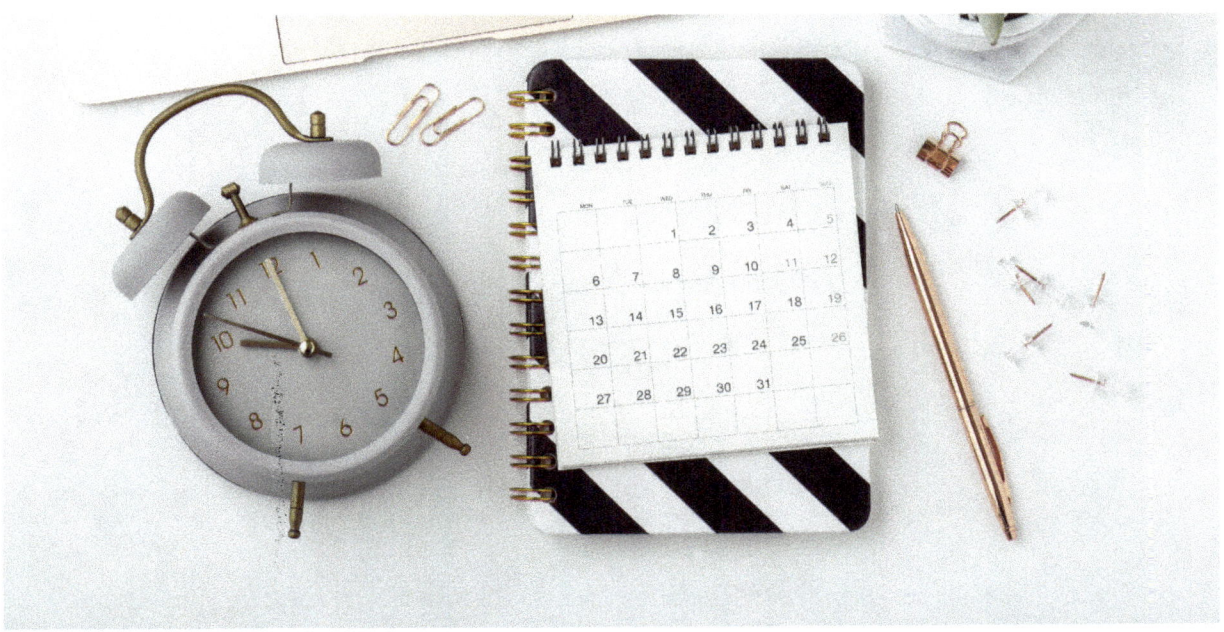

You 100% have to plan when (and where) you will eat.

Write yourself a schedule and then allocate times and then set alarms on your phone to remind you when to eat. Respond to the alarms; don't keep going until you're starving because you will make bad decisions.

Alarms and reminders will also stop you from naughty snacking and prevent dietary missteps.

You can decide what's best for you, and what fits into your schedule, and what works best for your body.

I do fasting and only eat between 11 a.m. and 7 p.m. I try and leave about 3-4 hours between eating so my body has time to process meals. After 7 p.m. I drink herbal teas and water but no snacking when I think I'm hungry but am just bored. This makes sure my mind doesn't play tricks on me and tell me I need snacks or treats or cheats.

Make sure you are eating enough. Don't under-eat, so that you're hungry an hour later. You also don't have to finish what's on your plate if you've had enough. It takes a while to get this right, but I'm sure you will! Also, reduce your portion sizes. I use a side plate or bowl rather than a huge dinner plate to keep my portions under control.

Eating Out

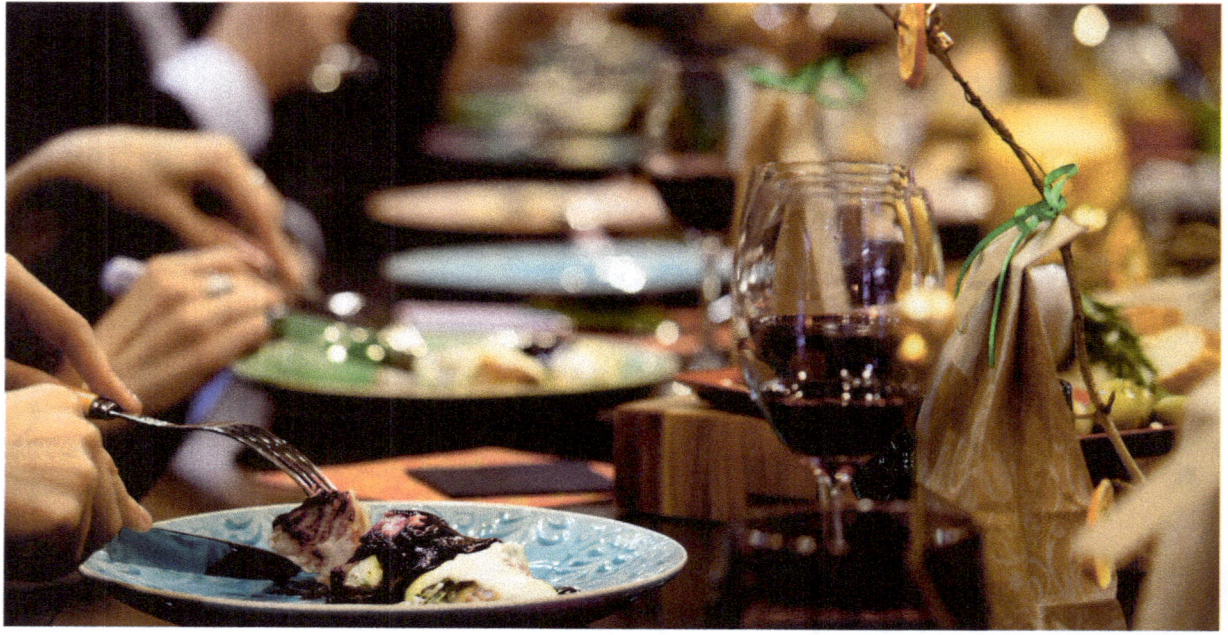

Please go and eat out. Go on hot dates, go meet your friends, and have a great time.

Life is way too short to deny yourself these precious moments.

But go in with a plan. You can almost always find a suitable SEXY option on the menu, unless, of course, it's at a dessert bar.

Go for the main course salad, choose something with protein and veg and have the fries occasionally, BUT NOT every time.

Dinner parties are great, but beware of arriving starving. I know this because I did this recently where I hadn't eaten all day, so when I arrived I hit the paté and crostini way too hard and then had regrets. Maybe have a light, high-protein snack or a protein shake, so that you are in control when you get there.

Dessert on the menu? Ask yourself if you HAVE to have dessert. You could probably say no and feel really accomplished afterwards. Opt for a coffee or a herbal tea instead.

I always have some dark 85-95% chocolate stash for moments when I have to have dessert.

Remember, every little bit adds up. Reduce your portion sizes and don't eat until you're stuffed.

Respect your body, it just does what you tell it to do. We ARE what we EAT!

Booze...friend or foe?

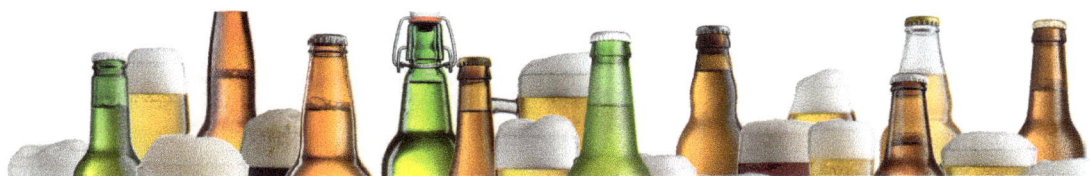

We just HAVE to have this conversation.

Alcohol should be enjoyed in moderation. It really shouldn't be part of our daily menu plan and yet society, culture and habits make it so easy to have a daily drink.

I'm not going to sugarcoat this. Alcohol is full of empty calories. Having a glass of wine or a drink every day is like having a cupcake every day, and you KNOW your body just can't deal with that, other than making it into hard-to-shift bulging thigh or belly fat.

"When alcohol is consumed, the body prioritises its metabolism over other nutrients. This is because alcohol is considered a toxin, and the body expends energy to process and eliminate it. As a result, the metabolism of other nutrients, such as fats and carbohydrates, is temporarily suppressed. This can lead to increased fat storage, especially when alcohol is consumed regularly or in excess. The accumulation of stored fat contributes to weight gain, particularly around the abdomen—a known risk factor for various health issues."

So, if you constantly ask yourself, 'Why am I still not losing weight when I'm hardly eating anything?' or, 'I'm eating healthy foods but can't seem to shake the weight or the centimetres,' it's no mystery.
It's the BOOZE.

It's fine to have a drink from time to time, but ask yourself why having a drink every night is so much more important than your health and well-being.
Alcohol is an addictive substance, so you will have to be strong and choose something else over that drink. It's called a bad habit, after all, so you owe it to yourself to break it.
So many people I meet say there is 'no way' they could live without a relaxing drink at the end of the day, but guess what? You can. You just need to choose to reduce its importance.
You only think booze helps you to relax because you tell yourself it does.
Try substituting an alcoholic drink with a FAKE drink. Make yourself a gorgeous bitters and soda with a slice of lime...bitters does contain some alcohol, so you're not going completely cold turkey. Or try iced teas or refreshing sparkling water in a wine glass. Your brain will associate the glass with a drink, but you'll be ditching the booze and reaping the benefits not only to your waistline and your wallet but also to your mood and energy levels. It's time to make a decision and take control back!

Rant over.
PS.
Yes, I love a glass of wine with a meal just as much as you do! But I choose only to do it when I have planned to treat myself. Makes it so special and enjoyable.

Travelling

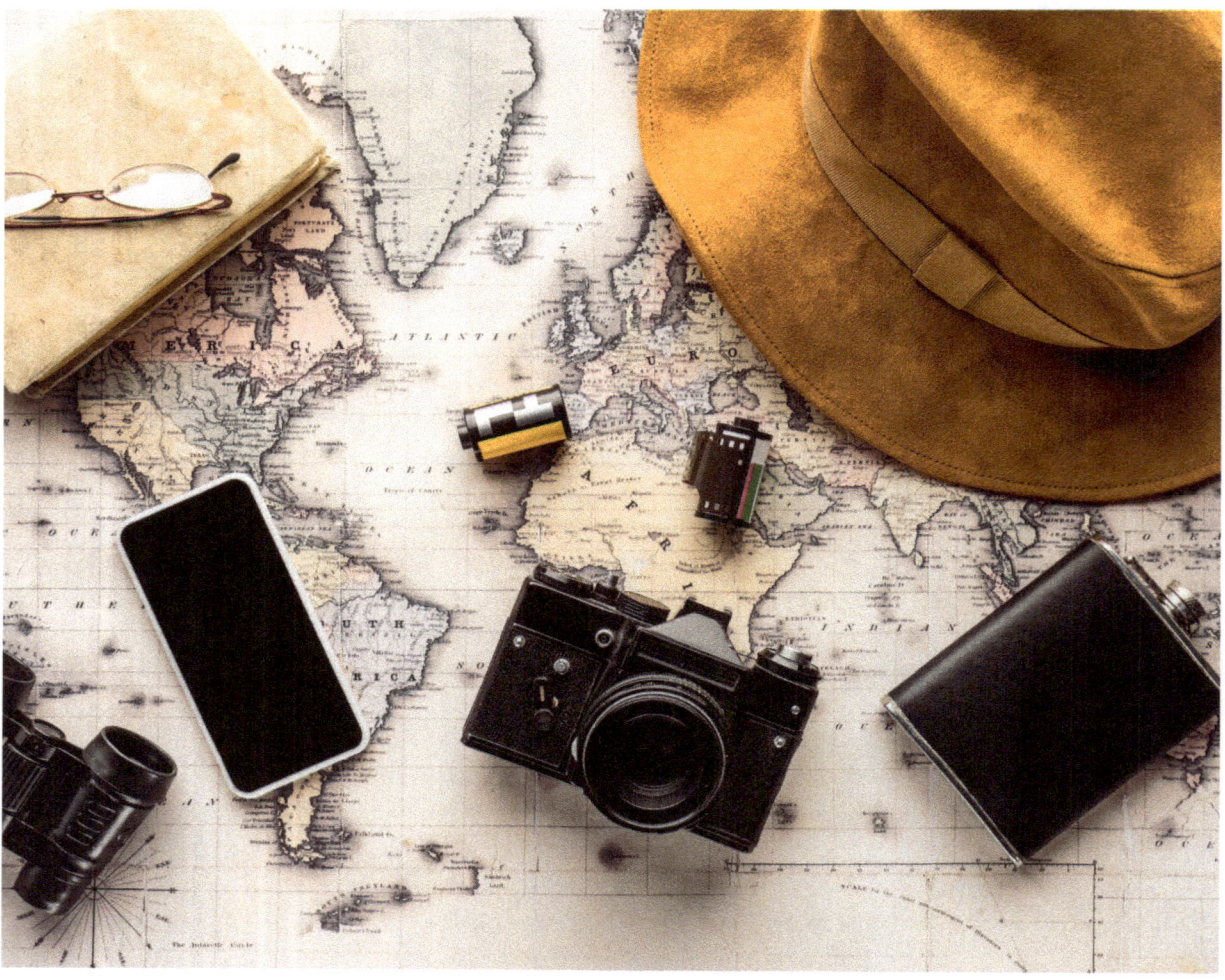

I love travelling, but what I don't love is coming home and realising I have put on a few too many kilograms.

Of course, it doesn't matter too much, you can fix the damage done in only a few short weeks, but here are some tricks I have learnt... and I keep improving them with every trip I take.

Have the treats, try the delicacies - that's what you have travelled vast distances for after all - but do it in moderation. Have half, share the other half, and keep it for later or tomorrow. Stop eating when you are full, especially when eating in restaurants every single day.

Massive main courses, buffet breakfasts and boozy lunches will start adding up, so eat with a plan. Have a few fix-it days in between where you eat lean and clean.

Do lots of walking. Hit the hotel gym. Those little bits of effort will save you from a distressing realisation on your return home that you went way too hard.

Snacking

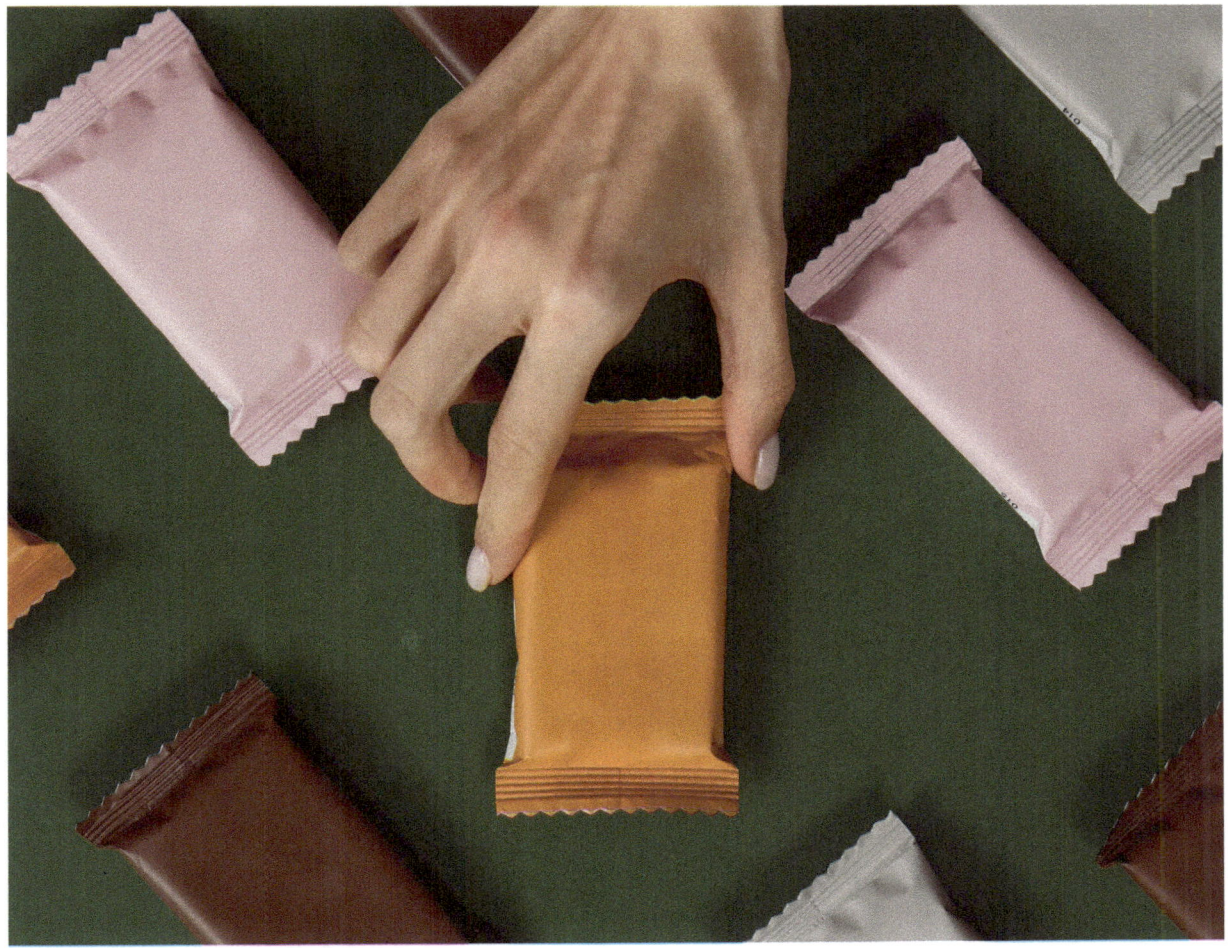

Snacks are great.
They can be healthy additions to your planned meals, such as lunchbox treats and small rewards.

But snacking can be dangerous. They have hidden calories, so just be mindful and have a big glass of water instead. Then come back later if you REALLY need the snack. Every snack you have will of course add up, so pay special attention to random snacking and try to train yourself out of comfort eating.

This is especially important late at night or when boredom sets in.
Ask yourself, 'Am I really, really hungry or just bored?'

I love to have my last meal of the day and then promise myself that if I feel like a snack later I will simply have a cup of herbal tea or a large glass of water.

If you just have to have something, opt for a high-protein snack and just have a small portion.

Hydration

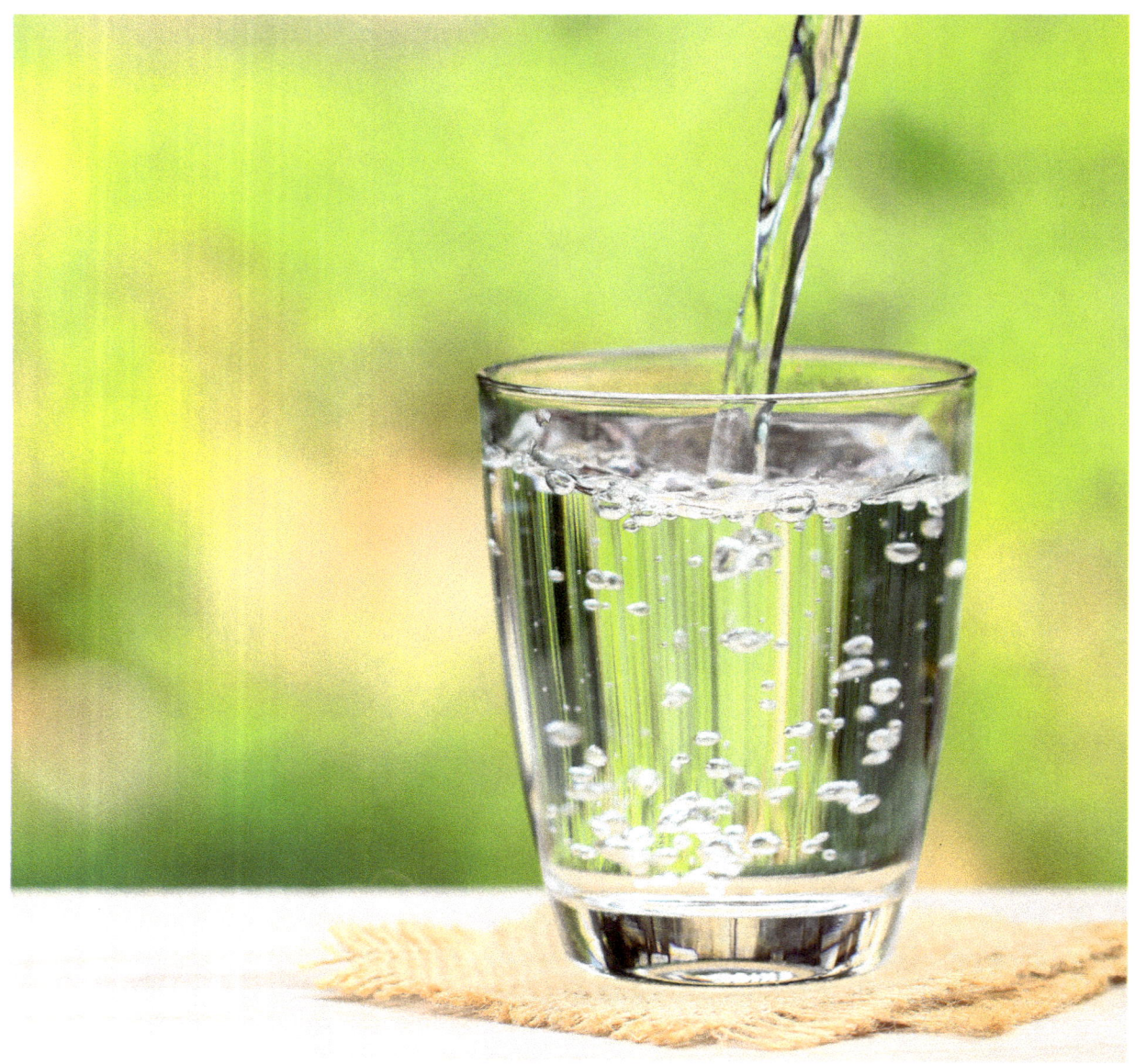

Hydration is important.

Try to drink at least two litres of water a day.
Get yourself a large bottle that you can fill up and refrigerate, and then sip on it all day.

Try drinking plain water or sparkling where you can.
You can also drink things like bitters, lime and soda, or sugarless iced teas instead of alcohol occasionally.

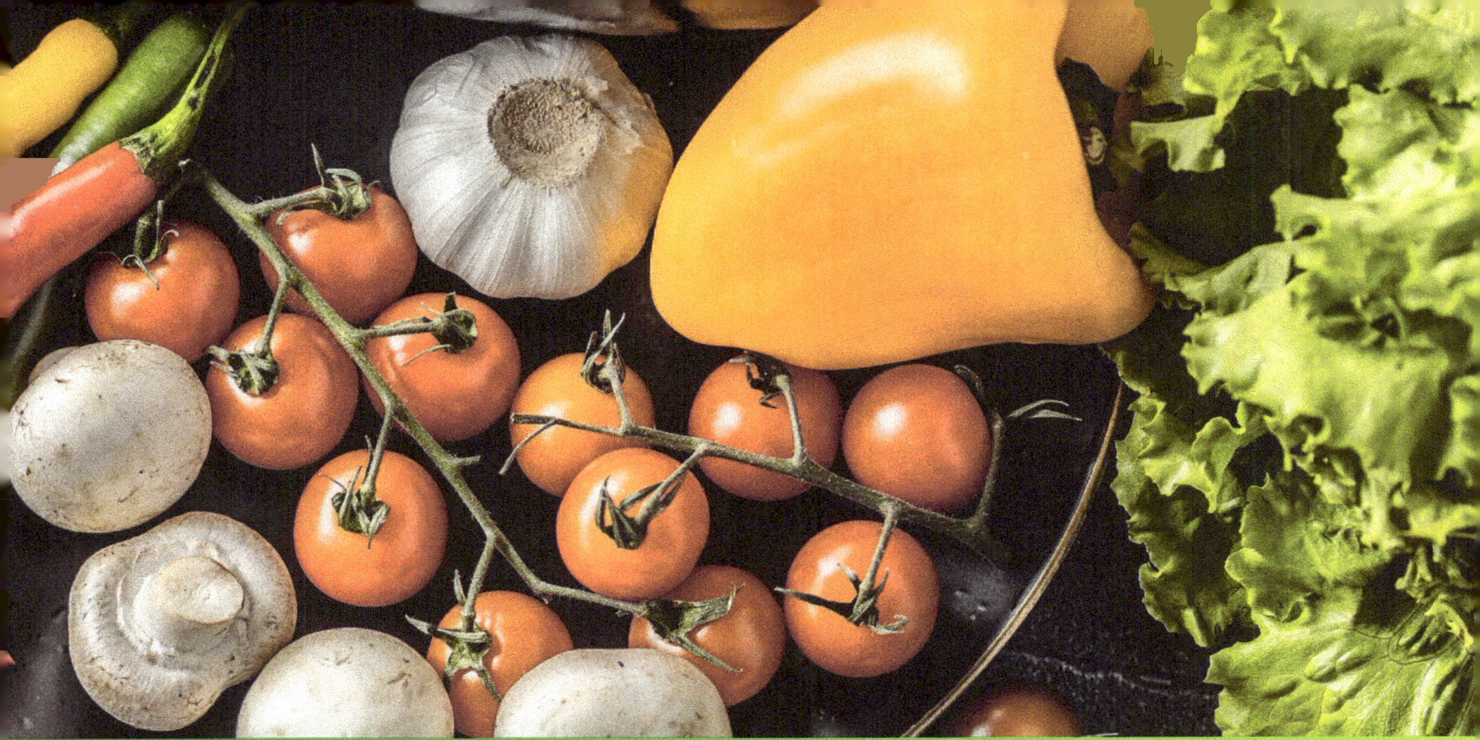

Shopping List

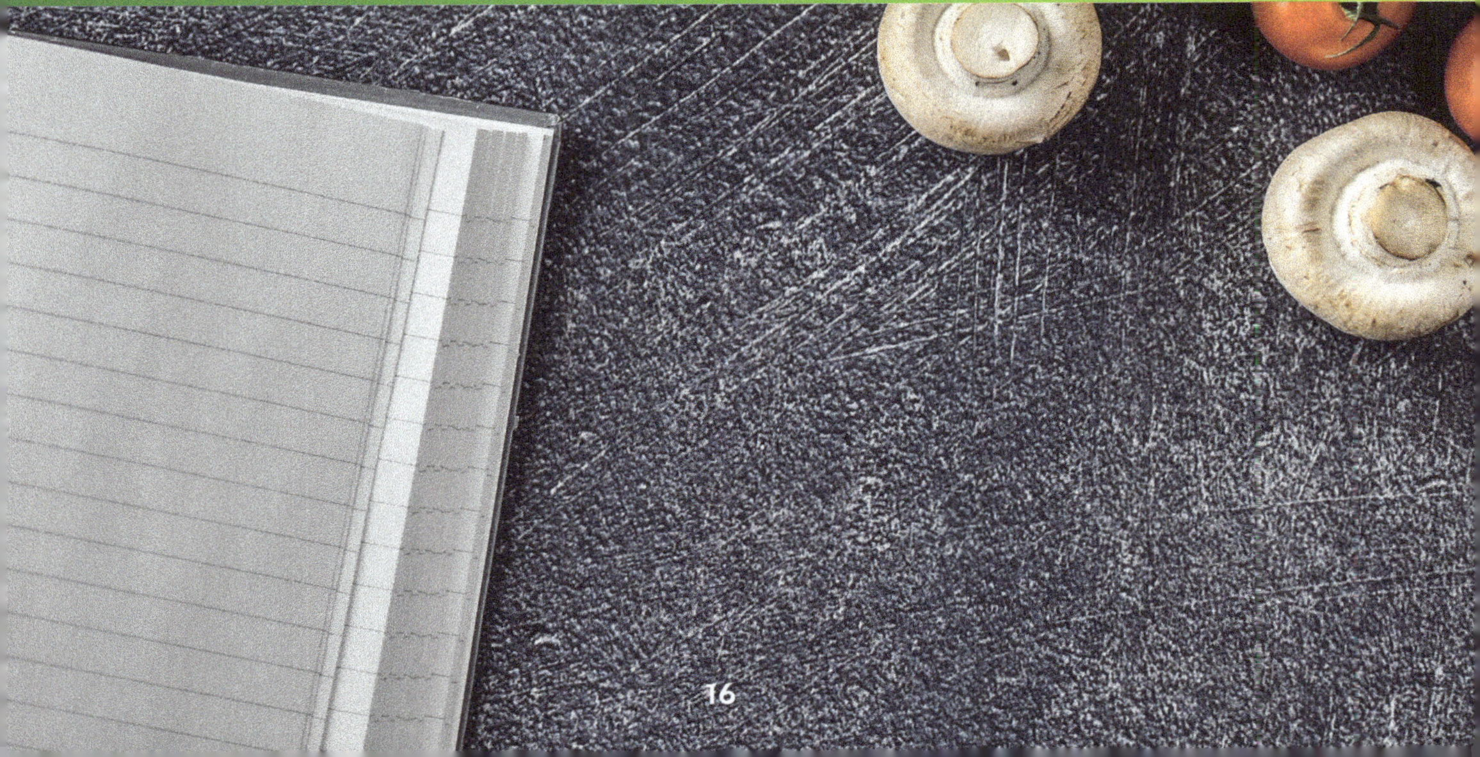

Fresh Produce & Pantry

Fresh Produce

Buy what looks good or buy on sale. Shop for the next three to five days. Quantity depends on how many in the family you'll be cooking for. This is based on a family of four so adjust as you need.

- 3 salad packs either pre-made or buy the bulk leaf pack
  (These are for the first few days so you don't have to prep. Once these run out you have your whole veggies to chop and use.)
- 1 kg tomatoes or 2-3 punnets cherry tomatoes OR Capsicum or both
- 1 head of broccoli or 2 packs Brussels sprouts
- 1 kg red or pink onions
- 1 kg sweet potatoes
- 1 whole red or wombok or green cabbage
- Also, get some avocados and your choice of lemons or limes
- 1 dozen large free-range eggs

Pantry

Check your Spices, Oils, Mustards, Vinegars etc for sexy dressings. We are also going to need some sweet treats!

- Tinned chopped tomatoes
- Fresh Cumin, Coriander, Paprika, Turmeric, Curry powder, Salt & Pepper
- Fresh Olive Oil, A Vegetable oil of your choice
- Mustard (grainy or Dijon etc.)
- Balsamic vinegar, White balsamic
- Kewpie or whole egg mayo
- 90% Dark Chocolate
- Cocoa, Cocoa Nibs
- Shredded Coconut
- Chia Seeds
- Almond Meal
- Vanilla Paste
- High Protein, Low Carb Protein or Whey Powder (check the side panel).
  We want high protein (75+%) & low carb (less than 8%) as a rough guide.

Fridge & Freezer

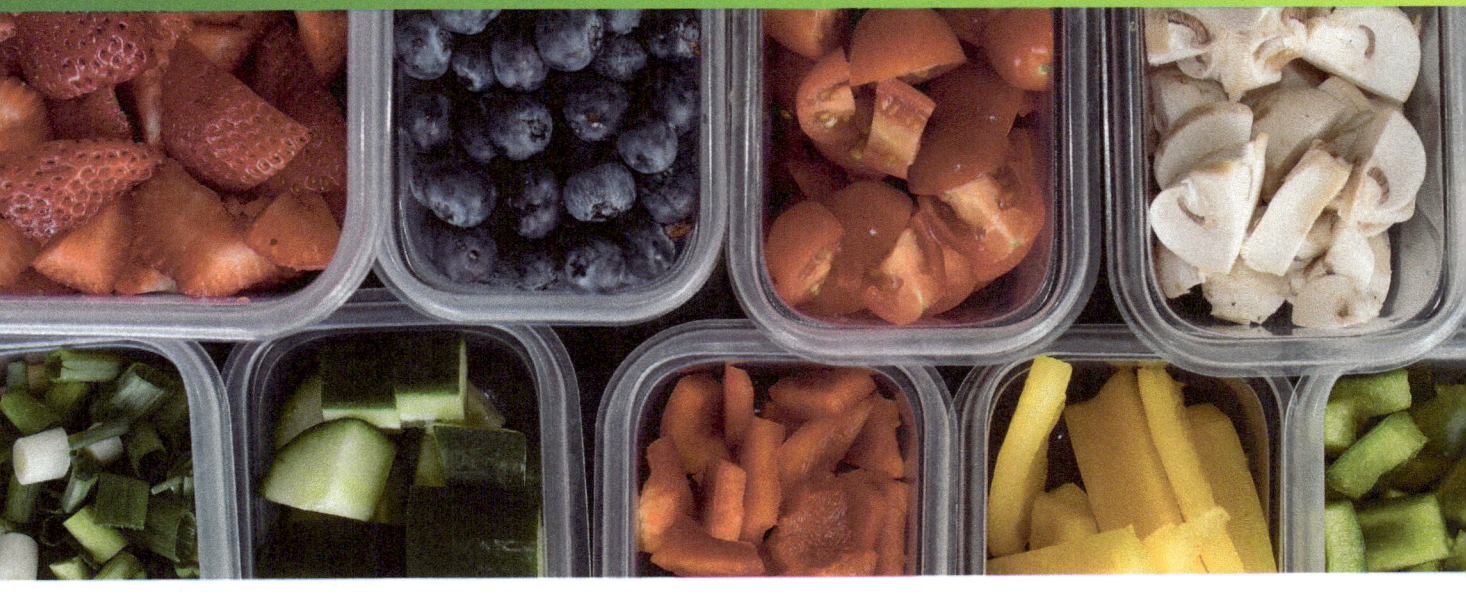

Fridge

We are going to mix and match these, so just get your favourites.
Get just enough for you OR buy for the family.

- Smoked Salmon
- Ham
- Fish Portions
- Chicken breasts/tenderloins
- Steak
- Mince
- Cream Cheese
- Feta
- Cheddar Cheese
- Plain Yogurt

Freezer

Even though I buy fresh portions of these,
it's handy to have frozen portions too, so stock up.

- Frozen Fish Portions
- Frozen Mince
- Frozen Chicken
- Frozen Veg (spinach, broccoli and others you enjoy)

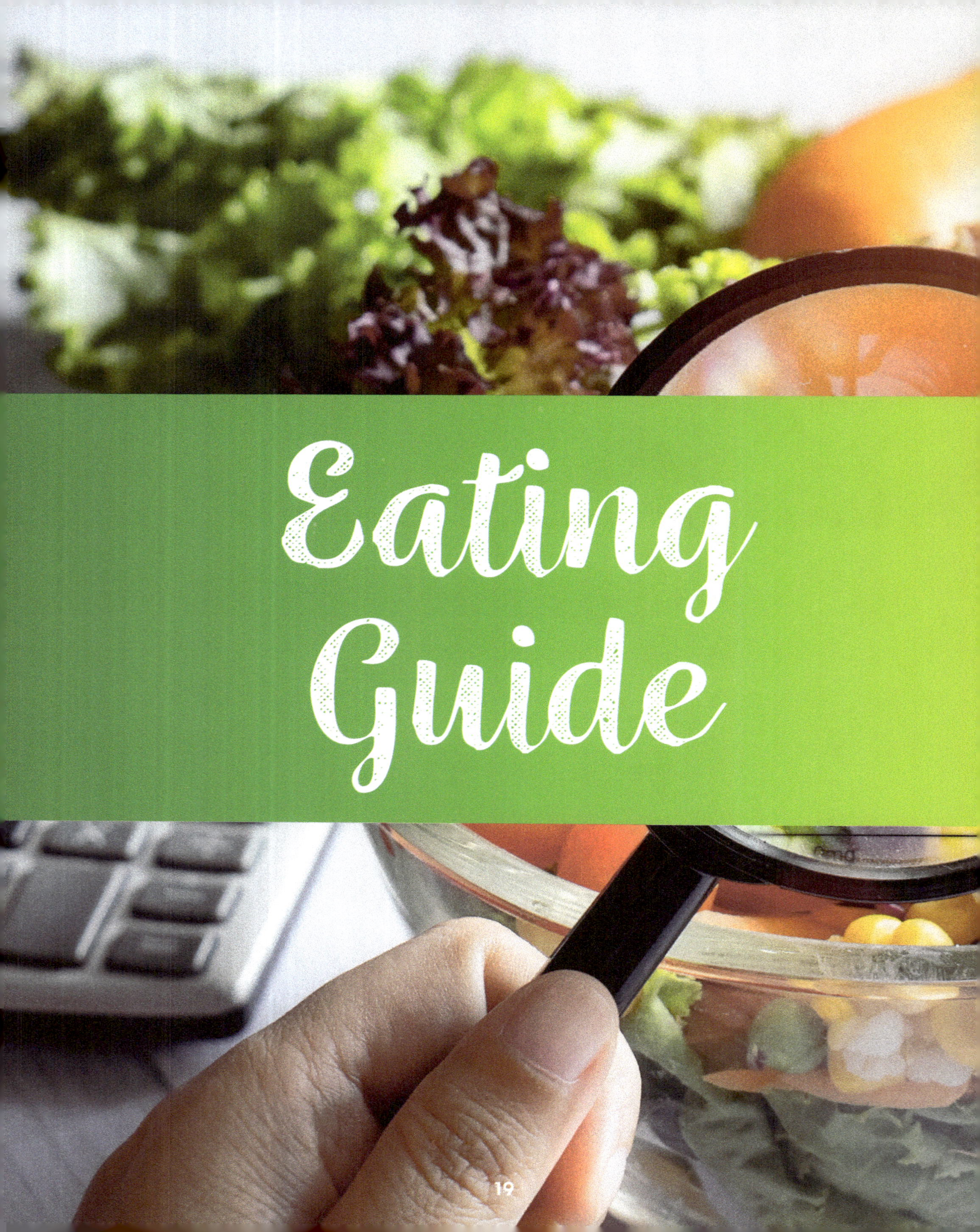

Eating Guide

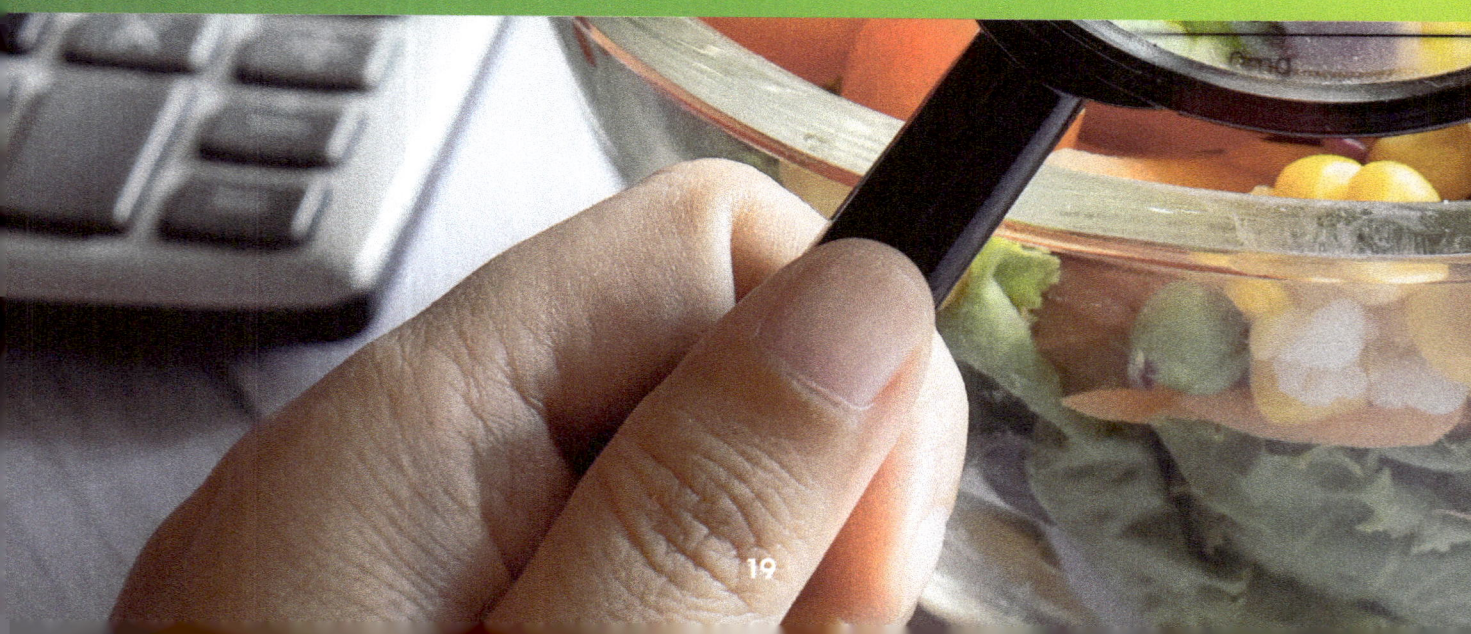

Easy Mix & Match Eating Guide

Breakfast Ideas

- 2 eggs, poached, boiled or scrambled on low-carb bread
- Berry Vanilla Chia Pudding
- Protein Smoothie
- Quickie Carb-Free Bread in a Mug
- Spanish Tortilla
- Omelette
- Sausage, bacon, eggs

Snack Ideas

- Boiled Egg
- 12-15 Almonds
- Cheese
- Wholegrain crackers
- Celery/Carrot sticks

Lunches and Dinners

Proteins

- Chicken
- Beef
- Pork
- Tofu
- Fish
- Lamb
- Legumes
- Some Cheeses
- Eggs

Veggies

- Zucchini
- Cabbage
- Brussels Sprouts
- Spinach assorted
- Kale
- Avocado
- Broccoli
- Capsicums/Peppers
- Tomatoes
- Cucumber
- Lettuce assorted
- Mushrooms
- Carrots
- Celery

Healthy Carbs

- Quinoa
- Brown Rice
- Pumpkin
- Sweet Potato
- Wholegrain egg pasta
- Lentils
- Chick Peas/Butter Beans
- Corn
- Grean Beans
- Peas

Healthy Plate Guide

FOLLOWING THIS SIMPLE GUIDE WILL MAKE PLANNING YOUR DAILY MEALS EASY.

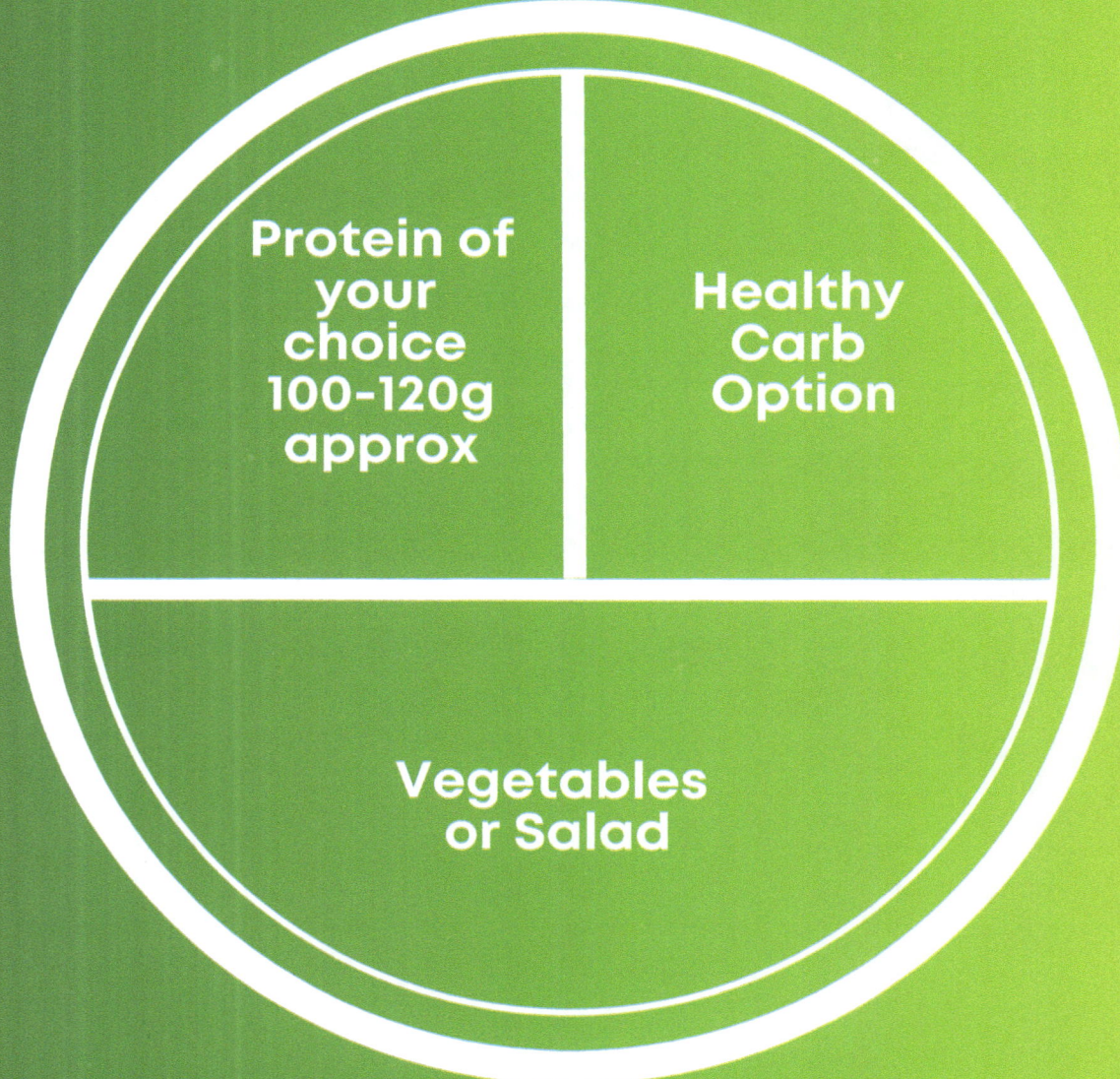

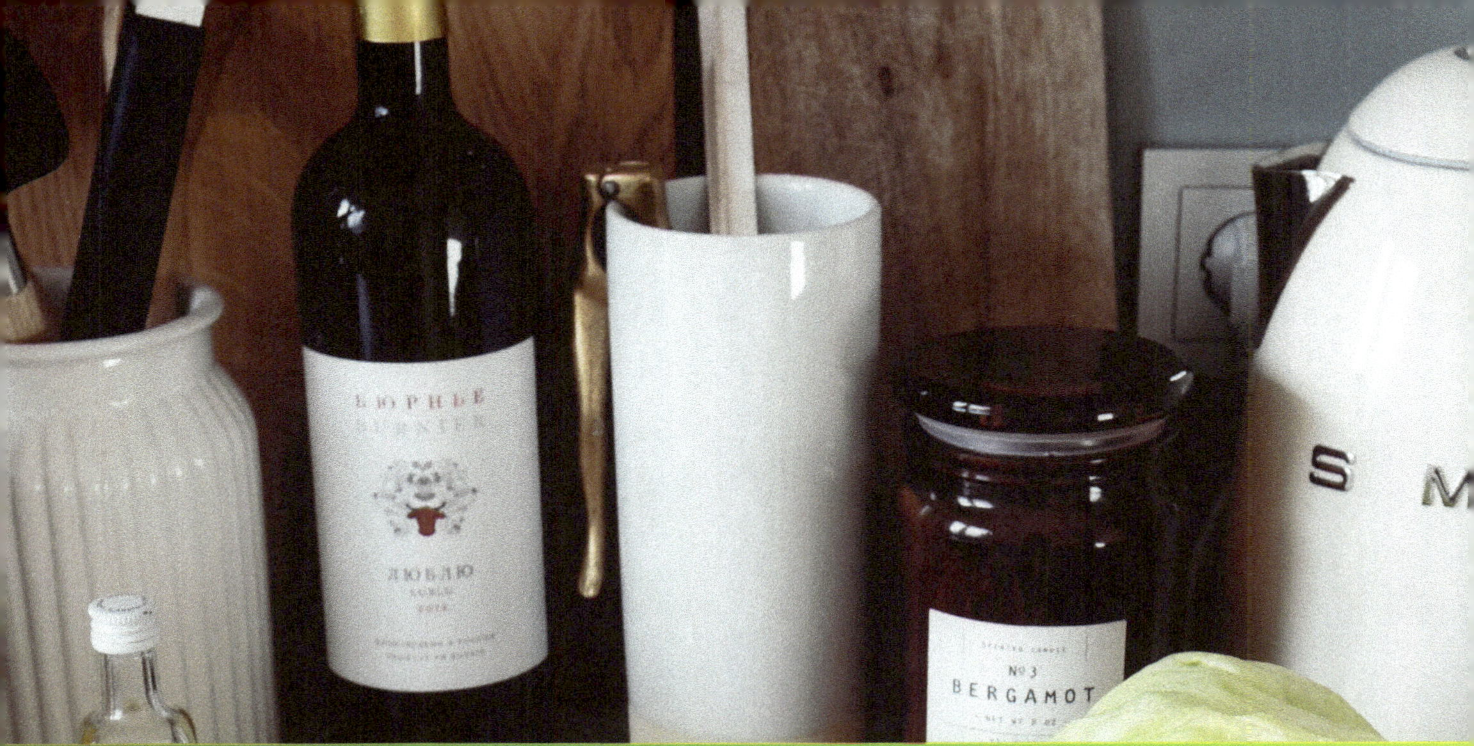

Recipes

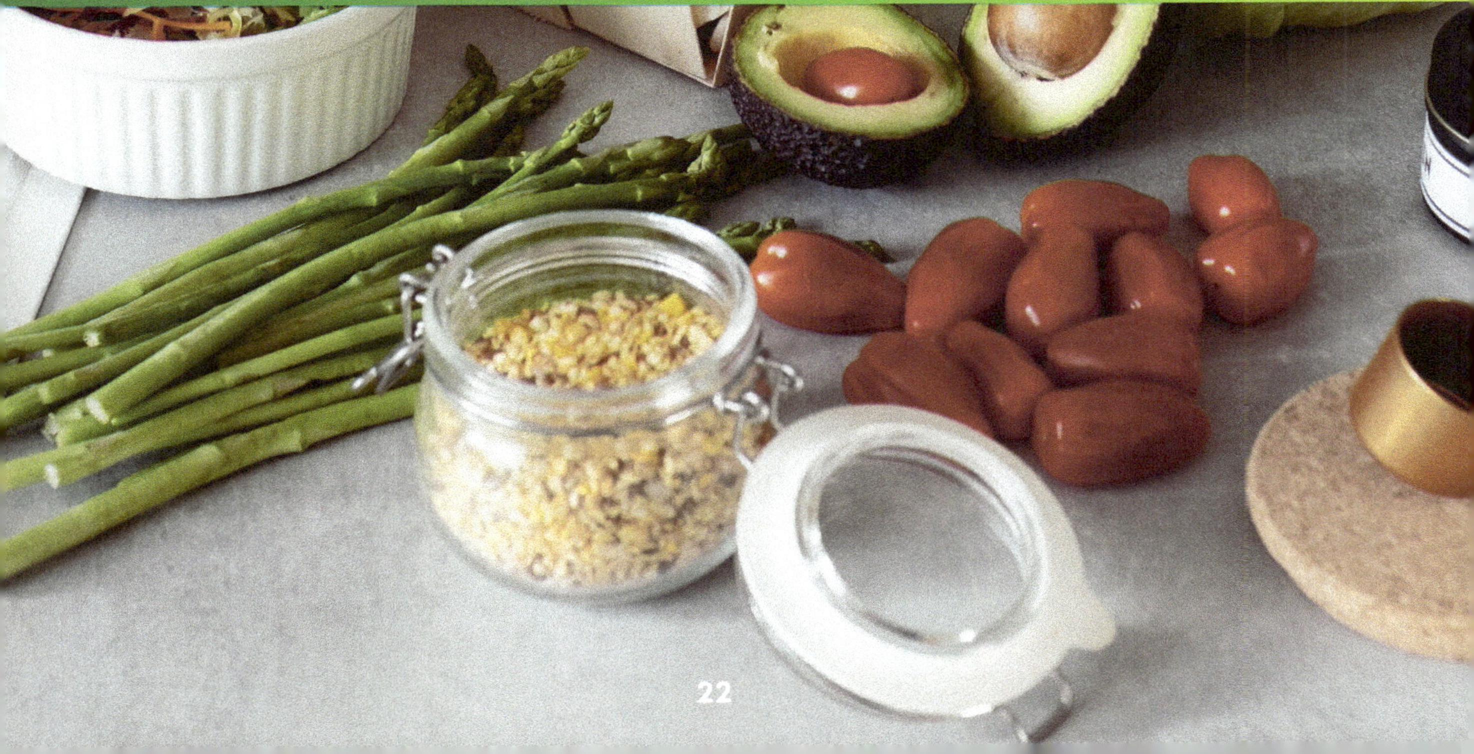

Recipes

Breads

- 27 — Quickie Carb-Free Bread in a Mug
- 28 — 5-Minute Keto Bread
- 30 — Seeded Wholemeal Wraps
- 31 — Seed Crackers

Smoothies

- 33 — Green Goddess
- 33 — Hershey's Hit
- 34 — Berry Bliss
- 34 — Mocha Mud
- 35 — Vanilla Nut
- 35 — Spiced Chai Latte

Breakfasts

- 37 — Beautiful Blueberry Pancakes (Keto or Traditional)
- 38 — Berry Vanilla Chia Pudding
- 39 — Bran Muffins
- 41 — Zucchini Fritters with Smoked Salmon & Cream Cheese

Egg Dishes

- 44 — Happy Sexy Quickie Eggs
- 46 — How to Poach an Egg
- 48 — Quickie Quiche in a Cup
- 49 — Easy Omelette
- 50 — Boiled Eggs with Bling
- 52 — Spanish Tortilla

Recipes

Salads & Bowls

- 54   Salad Nicoise
- 56   Beef Tataki Salad
- 57   Chicken Cobb Salad
- 58   Cajun Style Salad
- 59   Ultimate Broccoli Salad
- 60   Waldorf Twist
- 61   Prawn & Avocado Salad
- 62   Quinoa Salad
- 63   Joe Kools Chef's Salad

Bowls & Stacks

- 65   Miso Chick Pea Goodie Bowl
- 66   Buddha Bowl
- 68   Mexican Mince Bowl
- 70   Aburi Salmon Stack
- 71   Pimp Up a Tin of Tuna

Sauces & Dressings

- 73   Carrot Ginger Dressing
- 73   Asian Style Dressing
- 74   Vinaigrette Dressing
- 75   Best-Ever Creamy Kewpie Pepper Dressing
- 76   Make-It-Yourself Lemon Mayo
- 77   Nam Jim Dressing

Soups

- 79   Lentil & Vegetable Soup *with Creamy Curry Swirl*
- 80   Chicken & Vegetable Noodle Soup
- 82   Tomato & Basil Soup
- 83   Creamy Thai Coconut & Vegetable Soup

Recipes

Mains

85	Zucchini Carbonara
86	Zucchini Bolognaise
88	Vegetarian Stir Fry with Tofu
89	Baked Stuffed Capsicums/Peppers
90	Quickie Lentil & Sweet Potato Curry
92	Baked Stuffed Portobello Mushrooms
93	Truffled Mushroom 'Pizza' *with Cauliflower & Sweet Potato Topping*
94	Cauliflower Paella
96	Sexy Stir Fries
98	Sexy Roast Vegetables
99	Around the World Chicken Breast
100	Chicken Involtini with Sugo
101	Grilled Lemon Herb Chicken with Quinoa Salad
102	Pesto Zucchini Noodles with Grilled Chicken
104	Home-Smoked Chicken, Mayo & Mint Gourmet Snacks
105	Quick Durban Chicken Curry
106	Glamorous Chicken & Cream Cheese Balls
107	Sweet Potato Ribbons with Turkey Bolognese
108	Fajitas
109	Moroccan-Scented Mini Meatloaves *with Cucumber & Cumin Dipping Sauce*
111	Magical Moroccan Mince Stack with Pistachio & Date Gravel
112	Fish Tacos/Fish Bao
113	Thai Fish Cakes
114	Baked Salmon with Roasted Vegetables
116	Seared Crispy Skin Fish *with Pancetta Bark & Rustic Pea Mash*
118	Giant Tiger Prawns with Peri Peri
119	Tea Smoked Crispy Skin Salmon
121	Chicken Larb

Treats, Snacks & Desserty Treats

123	Keto Cubes
125	My Own Personal Choc-Lava Cake in a Mug
127	Complexion-Busting Bedtime Cocoa
127	Cheesecake Freezer Cakes
128	Cheats Protein Ice Cream
129	Complexion-Busting Chocolate Salami

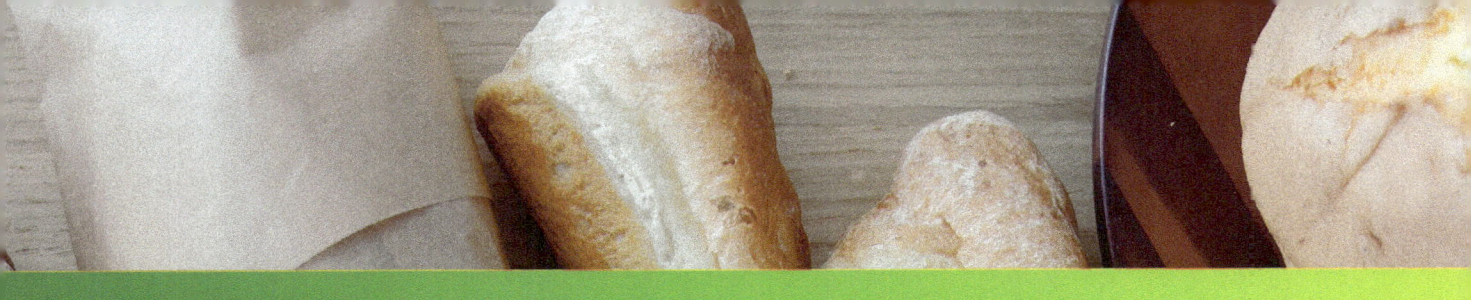

Breads

Let's get baking!

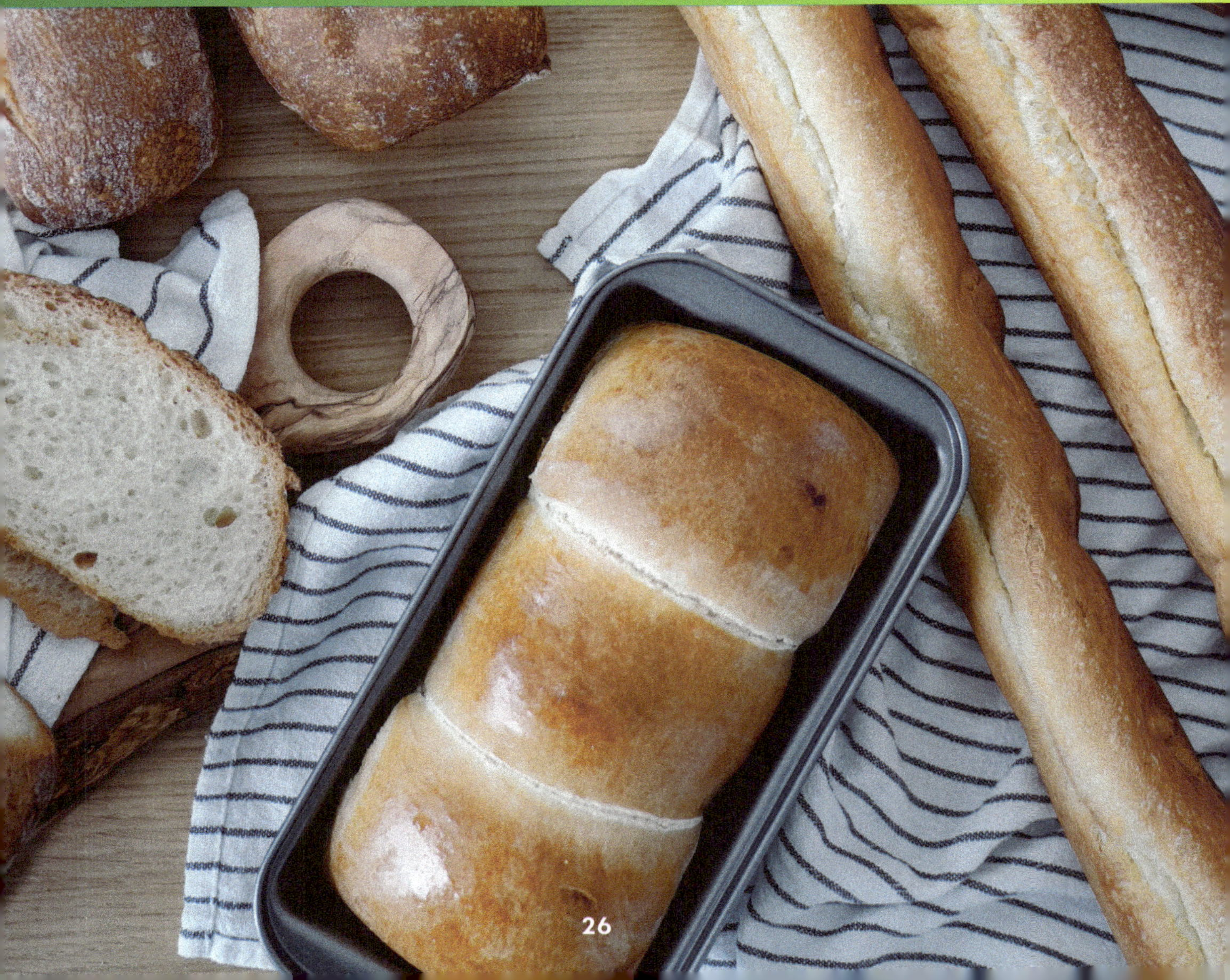

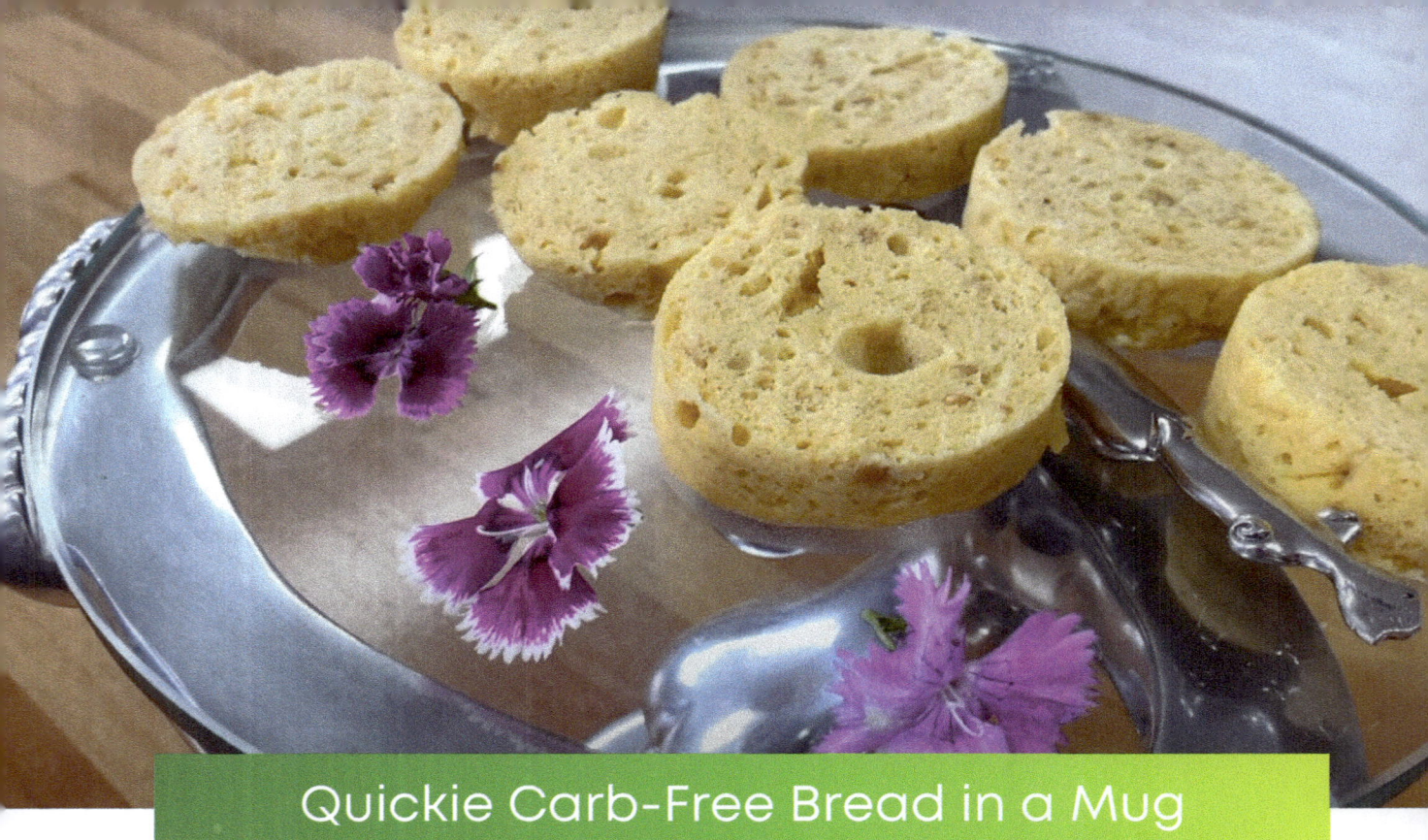

Quickie Carb-Free Bread in a Mug

SERVINGS: 1

INGREDIENTS

1 tablespoon crunchy or smooth peanut butter
1 egg
1/4 teaspoon baking powder
1 straight-sided coffee mug
Cooking spray

METHOD

Mix the peanut butter, egg and baking powder together by smashing them against the side of a small bowl with the back of a tablespoon. You will have to keep scooping the paste back in to bring it together. The thick peanut paste will take some squishing to blend with the egg and powder but keep going!

Put this batter into a greased coffee mug and cook in your microwave for ONE MINUTE.

Cool and then slice and have on its own or with your favourite spread, or as part of another dish.

Too easy. Too cheap. Too brilliant.

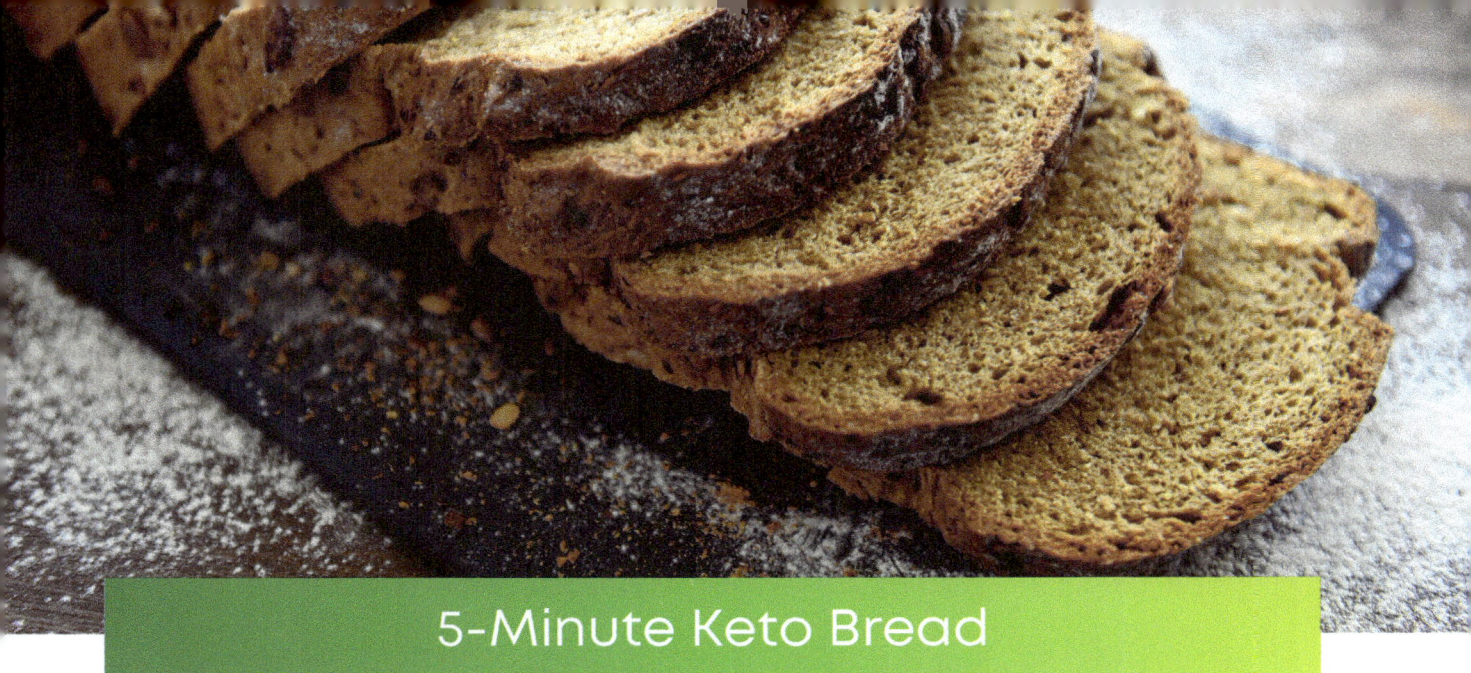

5-Minute Keto Bread

SERVINGS: 8 SLICES

INGREDIENTS

200ml water
200g almond meal
40g flax seeds *or chia seeds or LSA mix*
40g coconut flour
4 eggs
50g coconut oil or melted butter
1 teaspoon baking powder
1/2 teaspoon bicarb
1 teaspoon apple cider vinegar

METHOD

Simply place all these ingredients into a blender and blitz a few times until you have a smooth paste. Place into a greased baking dish and then bake at 180C for 15-25 minutes depending on the size of your container. I use two small pie dishes and then my cook time is 20 minutes, but you'll have to adjust depending on the size of your dish.
Once cooked, allow it to cool and then you MUST store it in the fridge to extend the life.
I slice mine when cold and then all I have to do is pop into the toaster to refresh.

Enjoy and please let me know what you think of this fantastic carb-free bread.

Happy Cooking

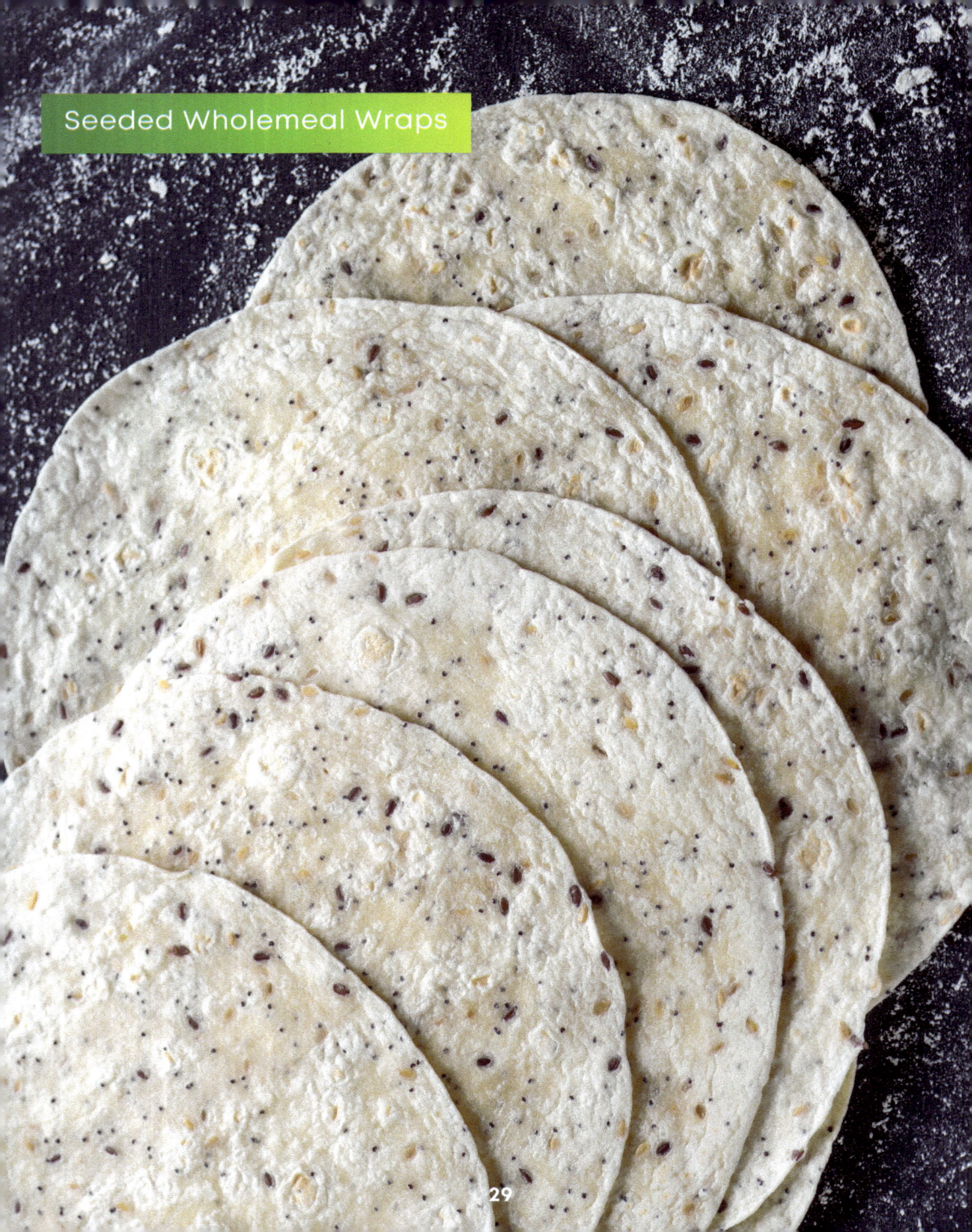

Seeded Wholemeal Wraps

Seeded Wholemeal Wraps

SERVINGS: 6-8

INGREDIENTS

450g bakers flour *or use half and half white and wholemeal plus 1 teaspoon extra flour*

1 tablespoon dried yeast

1 teaspoon sugar

320ml lukewarm water *or half water/half milk*

10g salt

30ml oil

Half a cup assorted seeds such as sesame, chia, linseed, sunflower

METHOD

Add the yeast, sugar and 1 teaspoon of extra flour to the warm water/milk.
Stir and set aside until the yeast has started to bubble and foam.

Place the flour and selected seeds in a large bowl and add the yeasty water mixture and oil.
Mix until it forms a firm dough.
Place on a floured bench or in a machine with the dough hook and knead for 5-7 minutes.

Place the dough into a greased bowl and cover it with a clean wet cloth, and allow to prove until doubled in size (at least 15 minutes on a warm day, longer if it's cool).
Remove from the bowl and divide into 8 -12 equal parts, depending on the size needed.

Roll out the dough to dinner plate size and then cook in a dry pan over a medium heat,
a few minutes on each side or until nicely browned.

Serve with the smoked chicken and salad as a wrap or as a dipping bread!
Top with scented olive oils, sexy cheeses, shaved prosciutto or the toppings of your choice.

"The only real stumbling block is fear of failure. In cooking, you've got to have a what-the-hell attitude."
— Julia Child

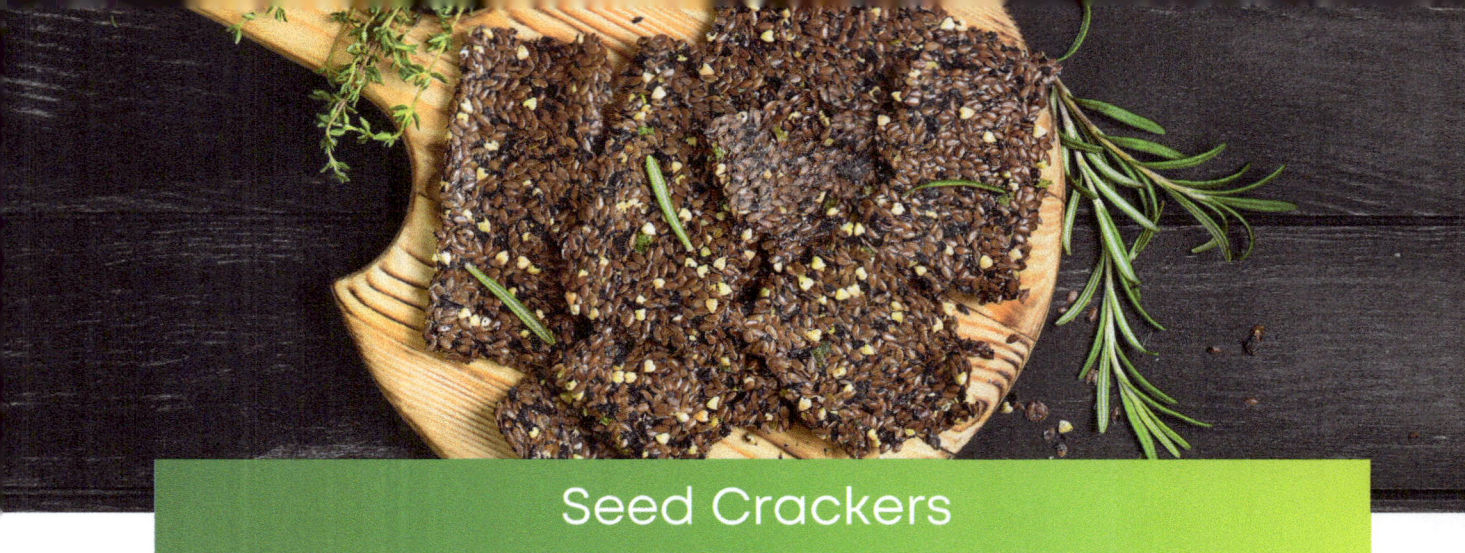

Seed Crackers

SERVINGS: 6-8

INGREDIENTS

1/2 cup sunflower seeds
1/2 cup linseed
1/2 cup flax seeds
1/2 cup chia seeds
1/2 cup pumpkin seeds
2 tablespoons psyllium husk powder
1/2 teaspoon salt
1/2 cup sesame seeds, black or white
1/2 cup warmed and melted coconut oil
1 cup boiling hot water

METHOD

Grease a large baking tray and line it with greased baking paper.
Preheat the oven to about 150C.
Mix all the dry ingredients into a large bowl and then add the hot water and oil. Use a strong spoon to bring the mix together. The chia seeds will activate with the hot water and will help form a gel.

Now press the dough onto the greased baking sheet and press it out into the tray. Pop another piece of parchment paper on top and roll out with your rolling pin to get these nice and thin.
Remove the top piece of paper and then bake for 35-45 minutes depending on the thickness, until they go crisp and the seeds smell roasted and fragrant.
Ensure you stand by towards the end if you have made these super thin, as the seeds could burn, so remove them when golden brown. Allow to cool and snap apart.

Perfect for cheese boards, snacks, salads, and soups where you need a sexy crunch.
Keep in an airtight container in the fridge or freezer to help extend the shelf life.

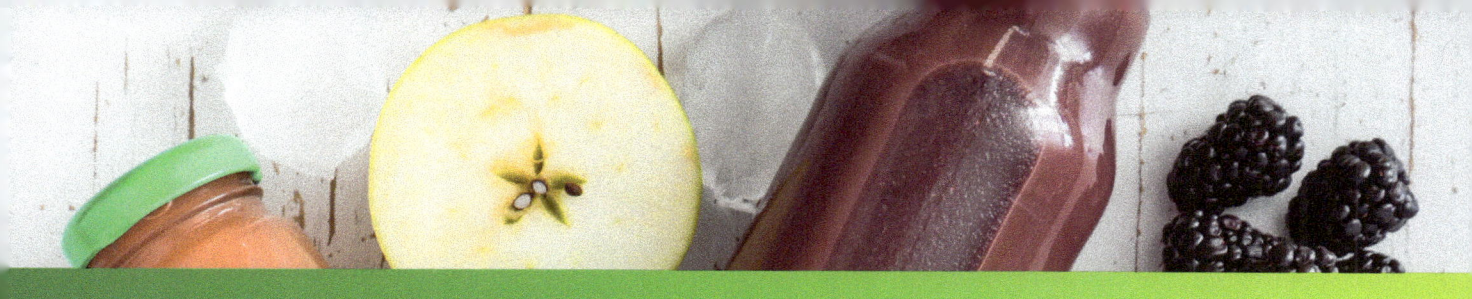

Smoothies

Single Serve Smoothies to Satisfy

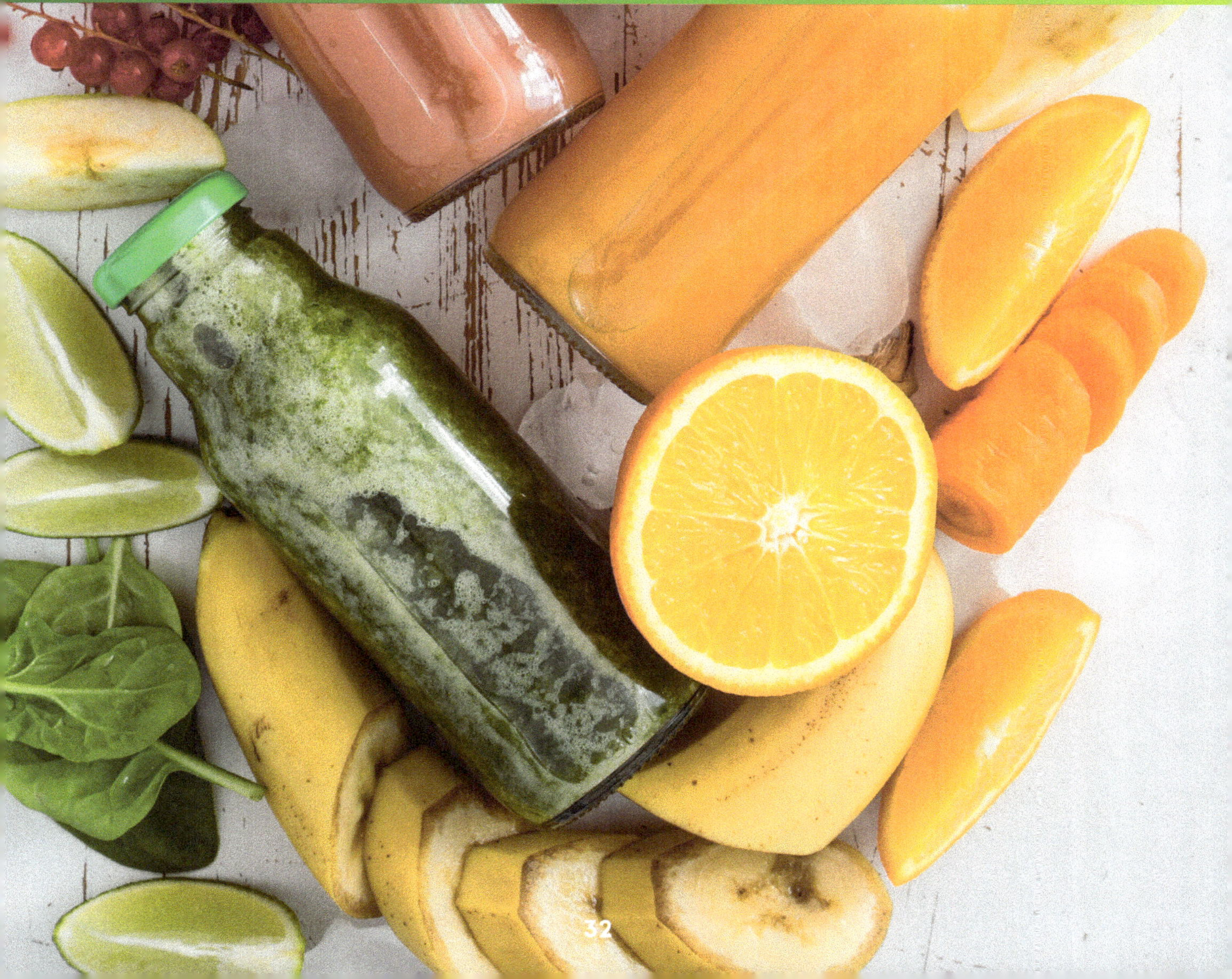

Green Goddess

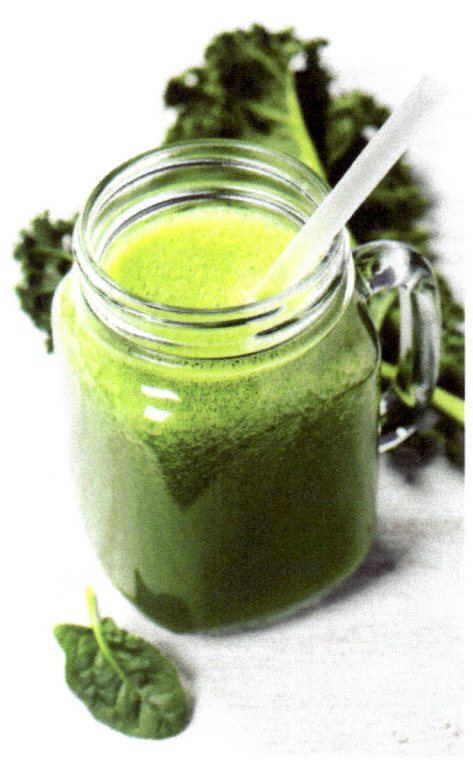

INGREDIENTS

1 x 75 ml scoop protein powder
100 ml cold water/coconut water
100 ml plain yogurt
1 cup frozen or fresh spinach
1/2 apple (or peach, pineapple or melon)
2ml vanilla extract or paste
1/2 cup ice
1 tablespoon fresh ginger

METHOD

Throw into a blender
Blend until smooth.
Bursting with nutrition and goodness.

Hershey's Hit

INGREDIENTS

1 x 75 ml scoop protein powder
100 ml cold water/coconut water
100 ml plain yogurt
1 tablespoon cocoa powder
1 large heaped tablespoon peanut butter
2ml vanilla extract or paste
1 cup ice

METHOD

Throw into a blender, blend until smooth.
I have this one when I need a treat.
Bursting with nutrition and goodness.
It is very decadent but will keep you full for ages!

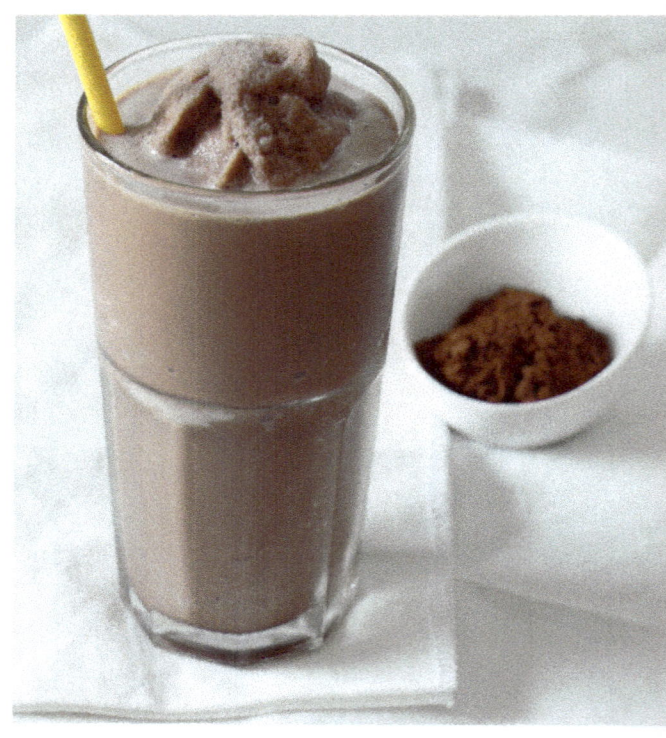

Berry Bliss

INGREDIENTS

1 x 75 ml scoop protein powder
100 ml cold water/coconut water
100 ml plain yogurt
2ml vanilla extract or paste
1 cup fresh or frozen berries
1/2 cup ice

METHOD

Throw into a blender, blend until smooth.
I love this gorgeous colour, feels like a little dessert for breakfast.
Use whatever berries you have available.
Bursting with nutrition and goodness.
Very decadent and delicious
AND will keep you full for ages!

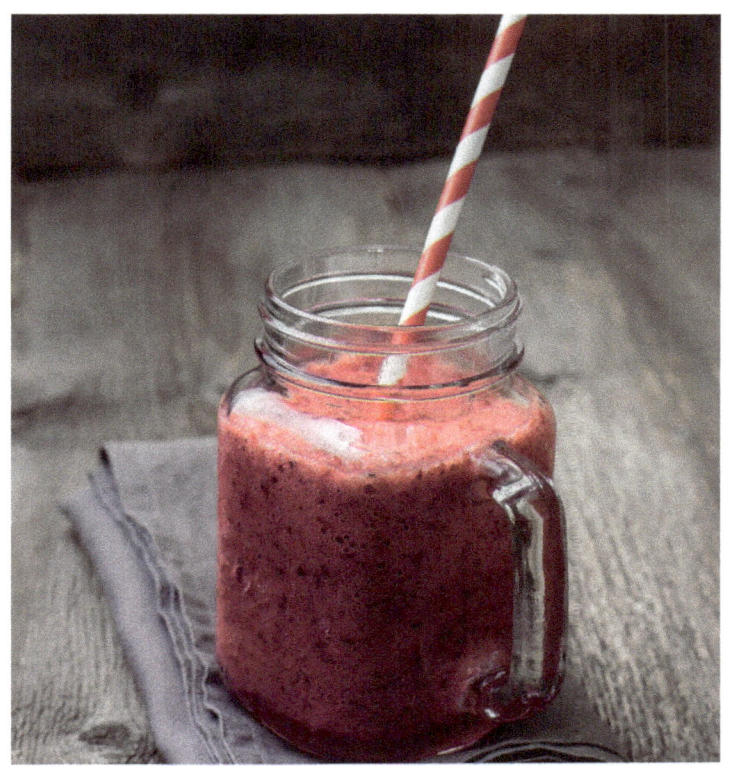

Mocha Mud

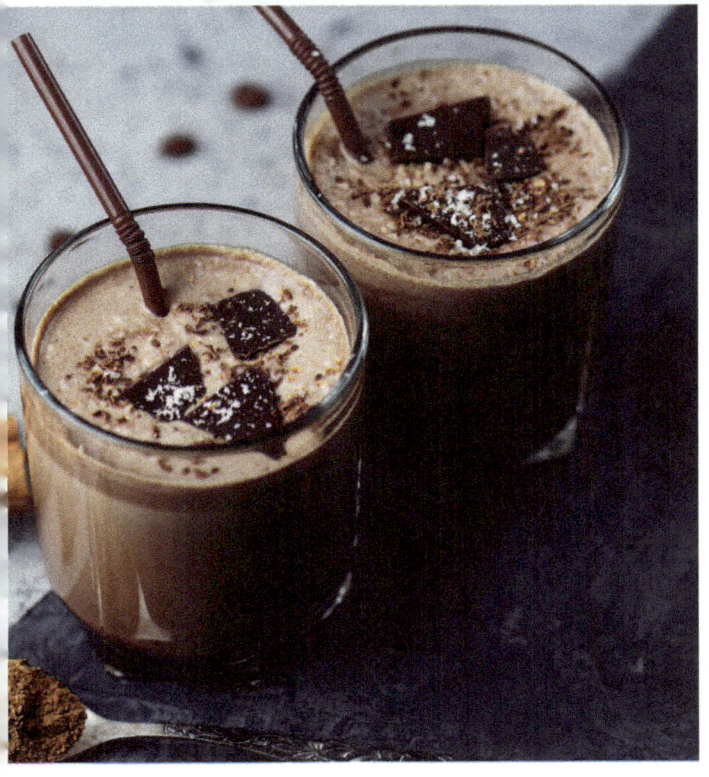

INGREDIENTS

1 x 75 ml scoop protein powder
100 ml cold water/coconut water
100 ml plain yogurt
1 shot of espresso coffee
or use 1 teaspoon instant coffee
1 teaspoon cocoa powder
2ml vanilla extract or paste
1/2 cup ice
1/2 teaspoon cocoa nibs to decorate

METHOD

Throw into a blender, blend until smooth.
When it is nice and smooth, decorate it with cocoa nibs.

Vanilla Nut

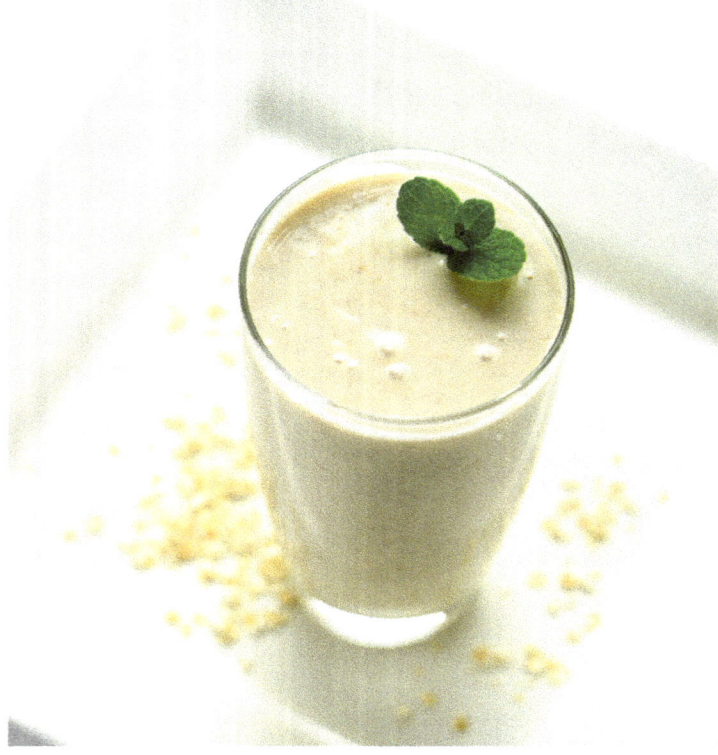

INGREDIENTS

1 x 75 ml scoop protein powder
100 ml cold water/coconut water
100 ml plain yogurt
1 tablespoon almond meal or use 8 whole almonds or hazelnuts
2ml vanilla extract or paste
1/2 cup ice

METHOD

Throw into a blender, blend until smooth.
I have this one when I need a treat.
Bursting with nutrition and goodness.
It is very decadent but will keep you full for ages!

Spiced Chai Latte

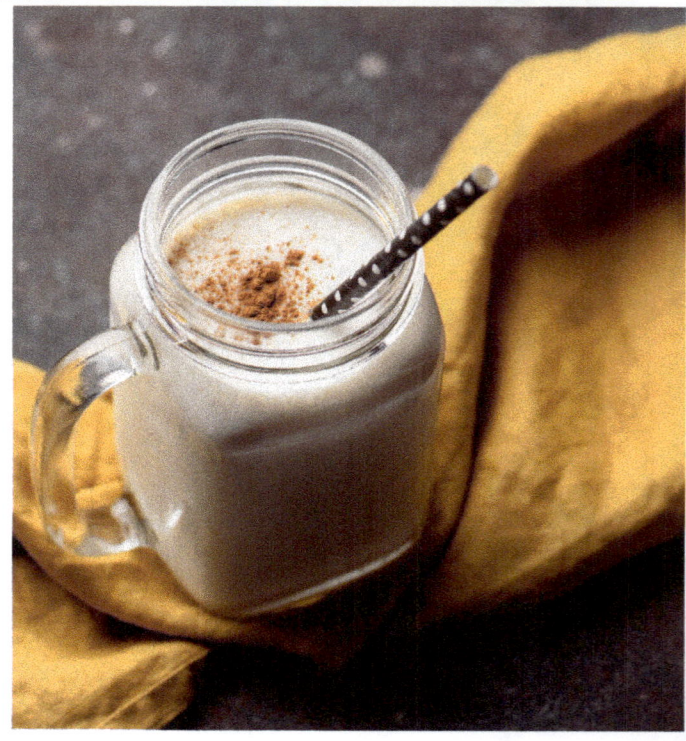

INGREDIENTS

1 x 75 ml scoop protein powder
100 ml cold water/coconut water
100 ml plain yogurt
2ml vanilla extract or paste
1/2 cup ice
1 shot of espresso coffee or 1 teaspoon of instant coffee
1 pinch cinnamon + 1 pinch nutmeg + 1 pinch cloves + 1 pinch allspice + 1 pinch cardamom

METHOD

Throw into a blender, blend until smooth.
This one is spicy and decadent, but still nutritious and will keep you full for ages.
Try your own special mix of spices and you'll have a delicious treat every time!

Breakfasts

Start your day right!

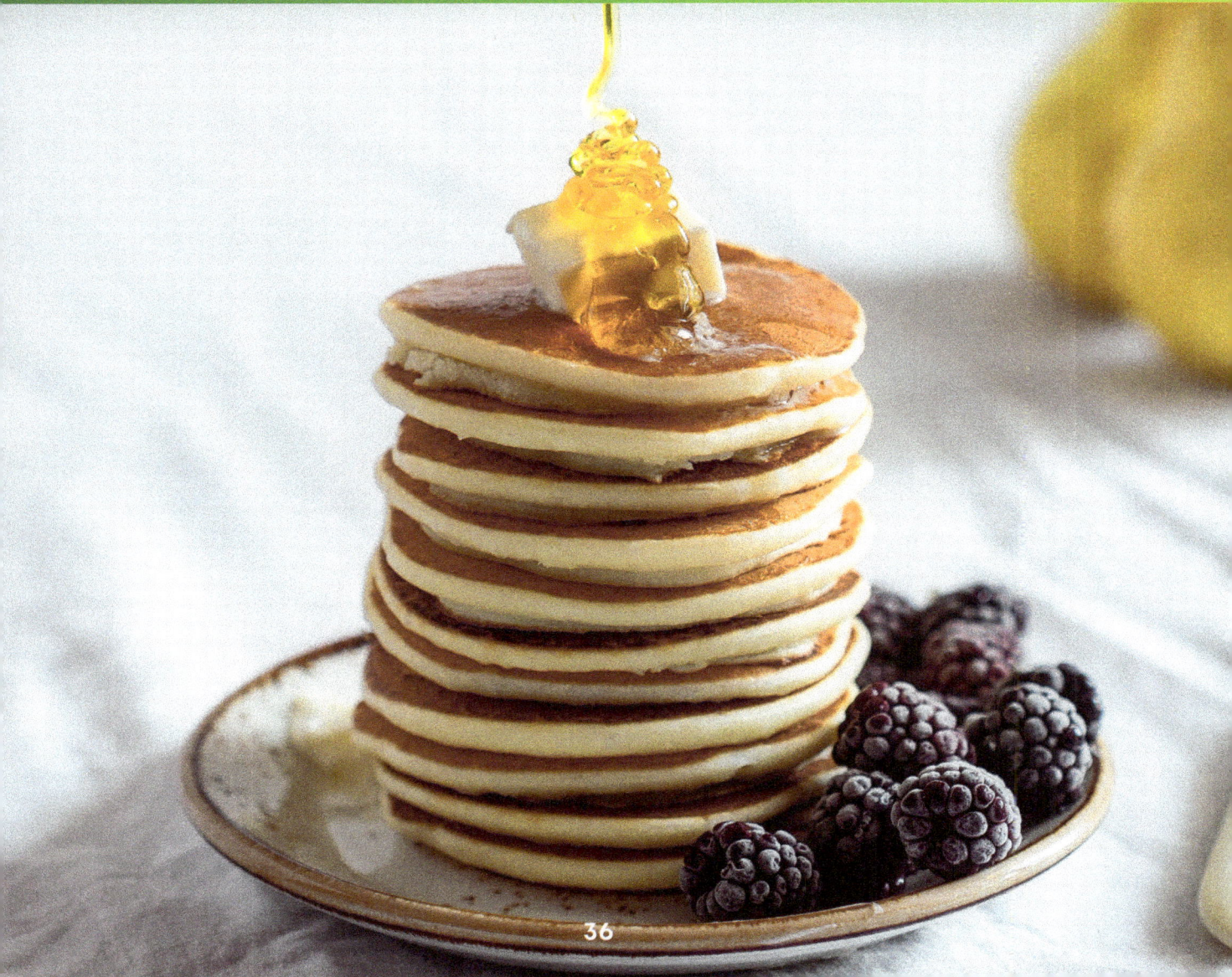

Beautiful Blueberry Pancakes (Keto or Traditional)

SERVINGS: 2-4

INGREDIENTS

BERRY PANCAKES

1 cup berries, diced if strawberry or just use whole for any other
200g plain flour
1 teaspoon baking powder
1 egg
300ml buttermilk or milk
50g melted butter
pinch of salt
5ml vanilla extract
2 teaspoons sugar (optional)
Vegetable oil or butter to cook
Syrup, cream or your favourite topping!

KETO VERSION

1 cup berries, diced if strawberry or just use whole for any other
200g almond meal
60g coconut flour or similar
1 teaspoon gluten-free baking powder
4 eggs
100ml cream
250ml water
50g melted butter or coconut oil
pinch of salt
5ml vanilla extract
2 teaspoons sweetener of your choice
Vegetable oil or butter to cook
Syrup, cream or your favourite topping!

METHOD

CHEF'S NOTE

For the KETO recipe, I decided to get you to make a bigger batch so you can have some leftover batter for a few days time. You can make this batter the day before your next beach BBQ or picnic, take it along and cook it on the spot!

Simply place all these ingredients together and stir, no need to complicate!
If you are using a NutriBullet or Food Processor, omit the berries and then stir them in once you have the batter. Or else they will puree…
Heat and grease a frying pan over a medium heat. Once nice and hot, pour some of the batter into the pan. Once a nice brown crust has formed, use a suitable-sized egg lift to flip these over.
Do the other side and then remove it onto a plate.
Stack and serve!

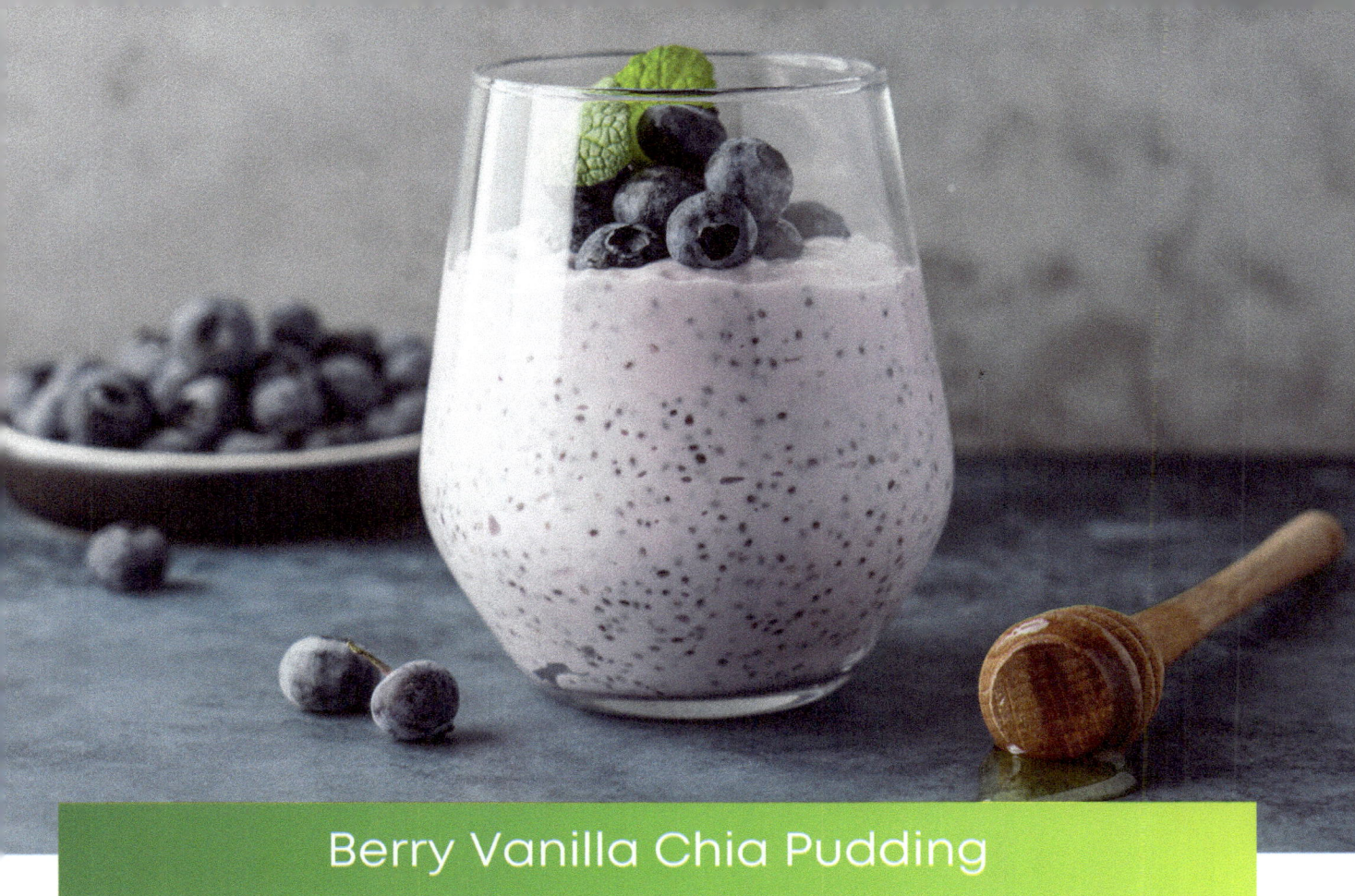

Berry Vanilla Chia Pudding

SERVINGS: 2-4

INGREDIENTS

375 ml coconut or almond milk
1/2 cup chia seeds
2 tablespoons honey or maple syrup
1 teaspoon vanilla extract or paste
1 cup pureed blueberries

METHOD

METHOD This is so easy to make, but it does need to be made at least 3-5 hours in advance.

Mix the milk, honey or maple syrup, seeds and berries and stir to combine.
Pour into ramekins, mason jars or cocktail classes and then set overnight in the fridge until they have gone thick and delicious.
You can also use other berries, I just love the purple of the blueberries; they look so decadent and pretty.
You can also add some protein powder to this if it will be your breakfast.

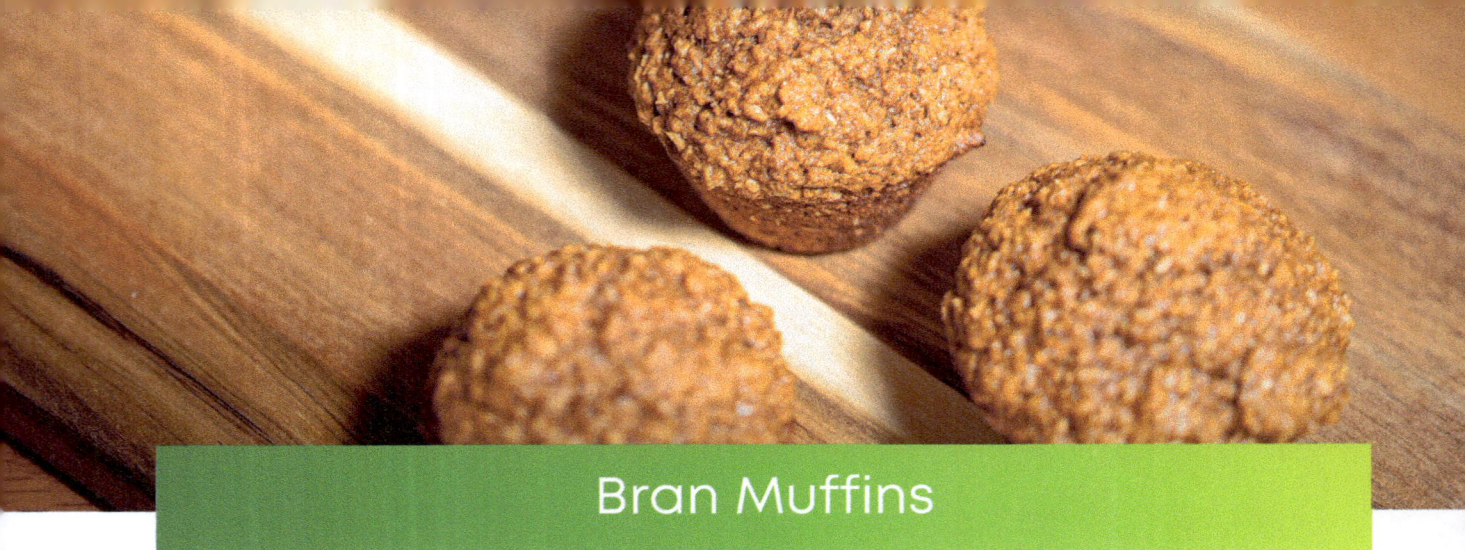

Bran Muffins

SERVINGS: 6-8

INGREDIENTS

2 eggs

1 teaspoon salt

1 1/2 cups brown sugar

2 1/2 cups plain flour, sifted

2 1/2 teaspoons bicarbonate of soda

2 cups milk

2 cups digestive bran

125 ml melted butter or vegetable oil

1 cup filling (see below for ideas – do YOUR thing!)

METHOD

Simply mix all the ingredients together until you have a smooth batter then spoon or pour into greased and floured muffin tins or terracotta pots.

Bake for about 10- 15 minutes at 180C until brown and golden.

You can then make them more special by adding a teaspoon of any of the following into the centre of the mixture in the muffin tin and mixing it in slightly before baking.

Strawberry yogurt

Marmalade

Assorted Seeds

Lavender and Honey

Blueberry

Apple and Cinnamon

Peaches and Crème

Banana Poppy ripple

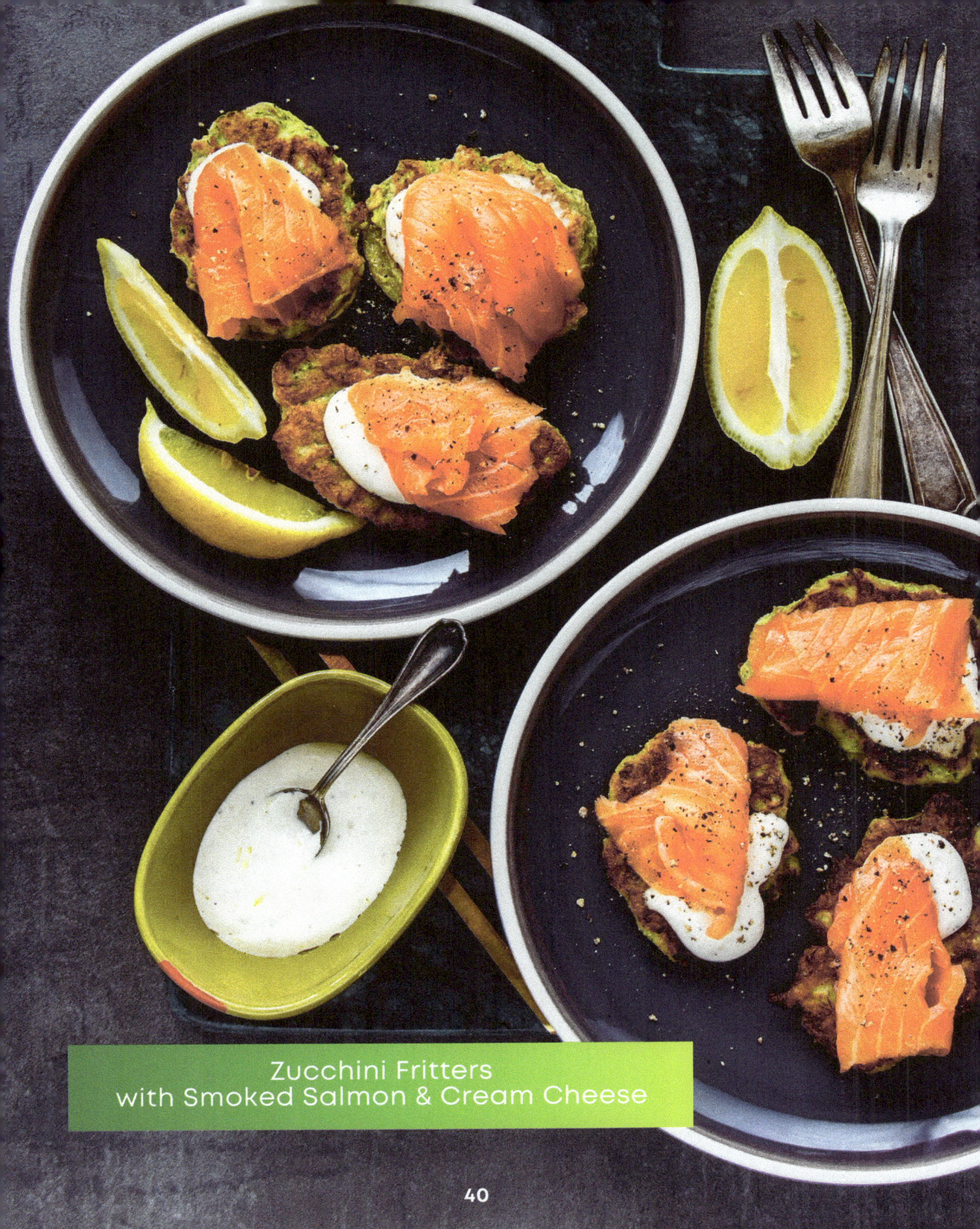

Zucchini Fritters with Smoked Salmon & Cream Cheese

SERVINGS: 2-4

INGREDIENTS

4 tablespoons cream cheese
1 pinch of pepper
1 pinch of lemon zest
2 eggs
1 pinch salt
1 medium zucchini, grated
3 tablespoons coconut flour, or plain flour or chickpea flour
1 teaspoon baking powder
50 ml melted butter or vegetable oil
30 g smoked salmon per person
A handful of rocket or tablespoon of herbs per person

METHOD

Combine the cream cheese, pepper and lemon zest into a paste.
Add the remaining ingredients and mix together until you have a smooth batter.

Grease a frying pan with cooking spray or a little oil; this will prevent any sticking later.
Get the pan hot over a medium heat. You can add a little more oil if you like.
Use a ladle or a spoon and make the batter into small round pancakes in your frying pan.
Allow the first side to brown and set - you will see bubbles forming on the top - then flip these over and do the other side.

Continue until they are all done, or keep some of the fritter batter until later.
Arrange on a plate and then serve with the cream cheese and the salmon,
with some rocket or herbs of your choice.

"I feel a recipe is only a theme which an intelligent cook can play each time with a variation."
— Madam Benoit

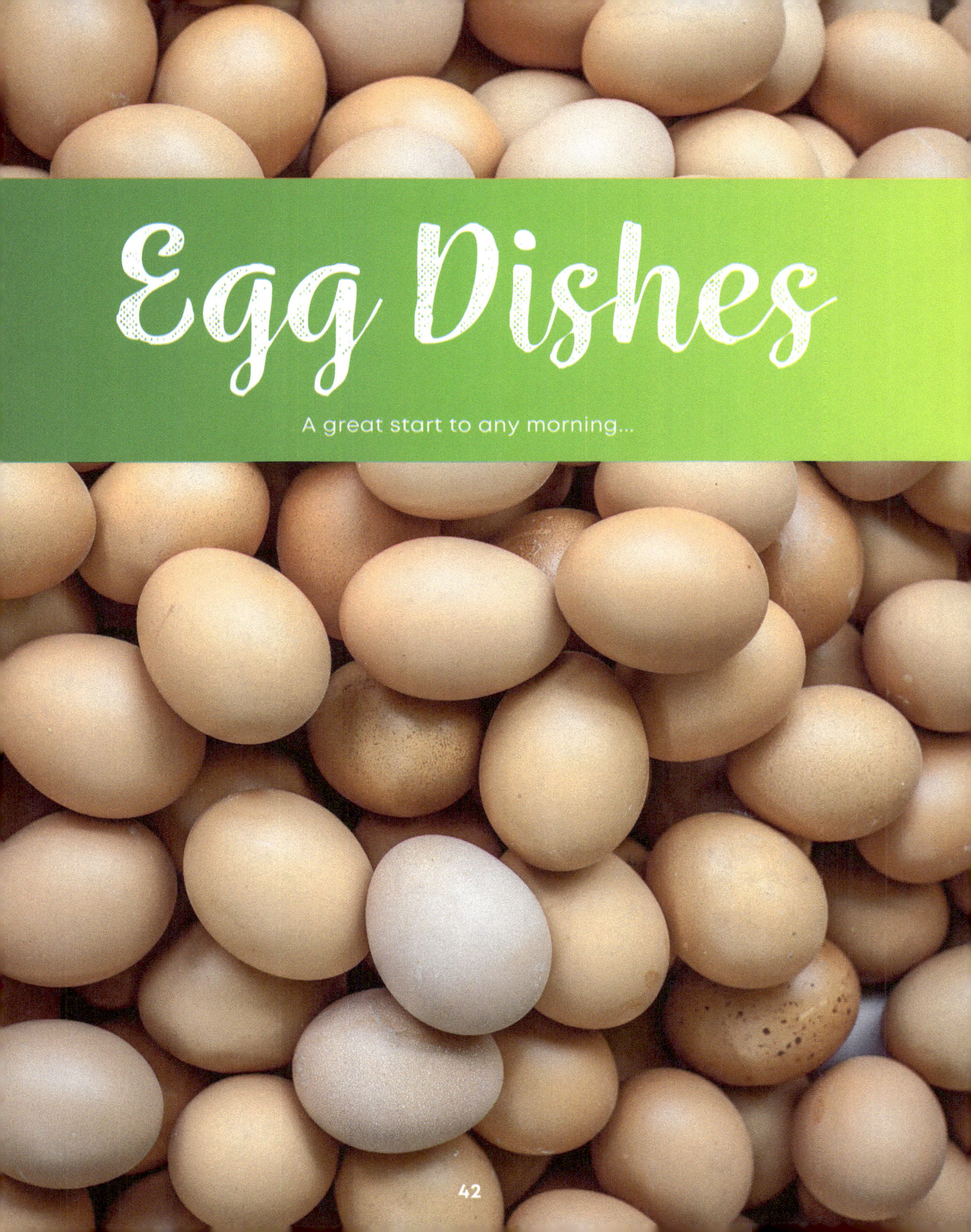

Egg Dishes

A great start to any morning...

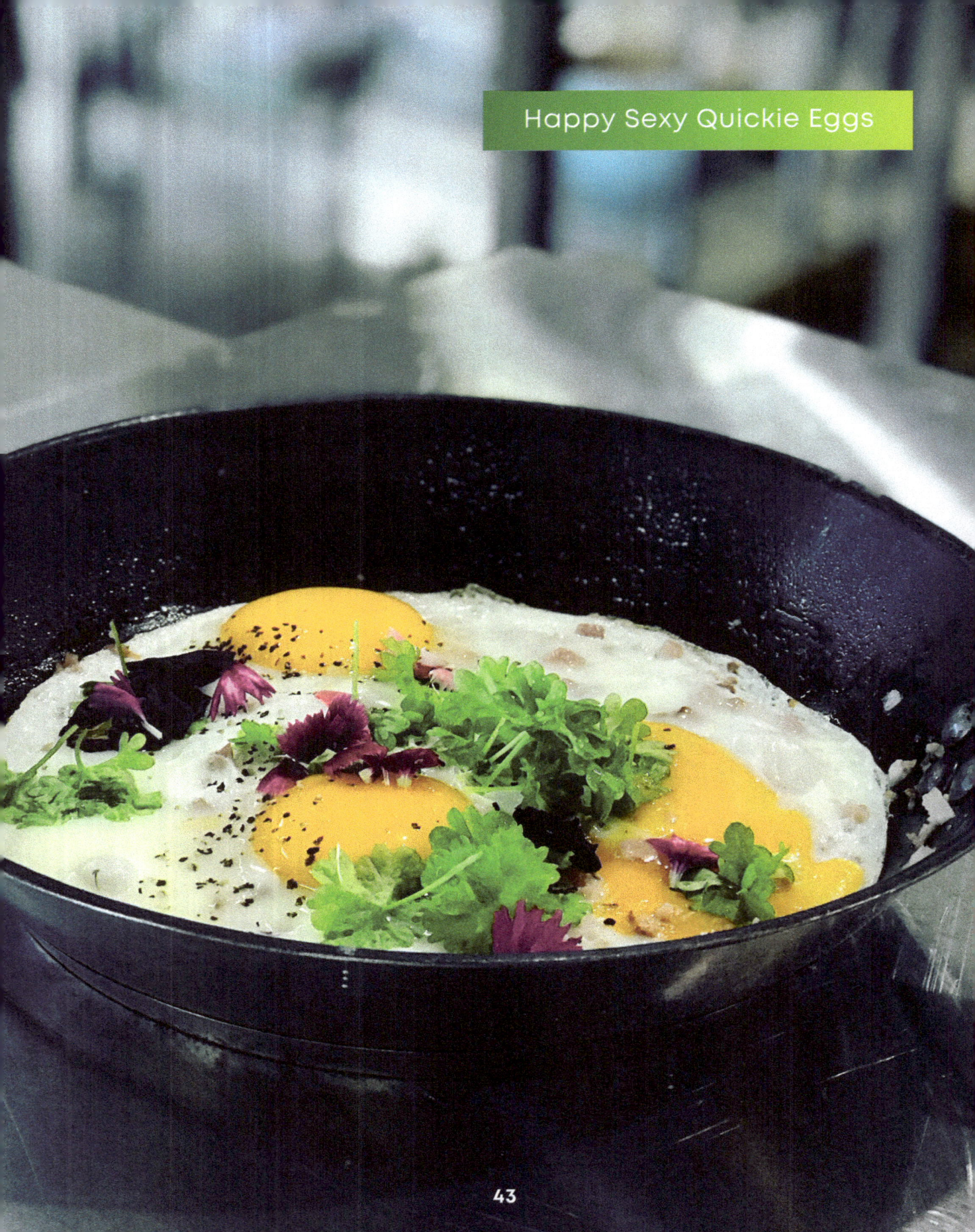

Happy Sexy Quickie Eggs

Happy Sexy Quickie Eggs

SERVINGS: 2

INGREDIENTS

Vegetable oil or cooking spray (not olive oil)
2 tablespoons chopped/diced bacon
OR Prosciutto/Pancetta OR Speck OR chorizo sausage OR mushrooms (you choose)
2 tablespoons chopped onions
OR Spinach OR spring onion OR zucchini OR tomato
3-4 fresh free-range eggs
1 pinch of pepper to season
1 tablespoon grated cheddar
Pecorino or Parmesan (optional)
Drizzle of truffle oil, and extra virgin olive oil (optional)

METHOD

In my quest for the laziest YET sexiest eggs, this has become one of my best inventions.
Almost a cross between an omelette and a fried egg - but the best of both!
Omelettes have the privilege of having a filling to make them a bit sexier.
Fried eggs are okay, but the large expanse of tasteless egg white is just not my favourite.
With this recipe, the white will be loaded with amazing flavour, colour and texture and will look ten bucks more expensive. Also, unless you have a fabulous pan, omelettes can make your language very bad when they stick and break and just don't turn out. Literally.
So, try my happy eggs, you can change the 'filling' to whatever you like.
I'll give you a few ideas and let you happy egg all by yourself! Enjoy.

You will need a small to medium frying pan with a lid for this recipe.
Heat and grease the frying pan well with the cooking spray. You DO NOT want to underdo the oiling and risk all your ingredients sticking. Place the diced bacon *(or speck, chorizo or mushrooms)* in the pan and let them go crisp and brown and flavoursome. Add the second ingredient *(onion, spring onion or zucchini)* and cook while stirring for about a minute until soft.
Now spread it evenly around the pan.
Crack the eggs over this deliciousness and then turn the heat to medium, put the lid on the pan and let those eggs cook through to the doneness you like: soft, medium or hard.
Season with pepper, oil, and it's ready to serve!

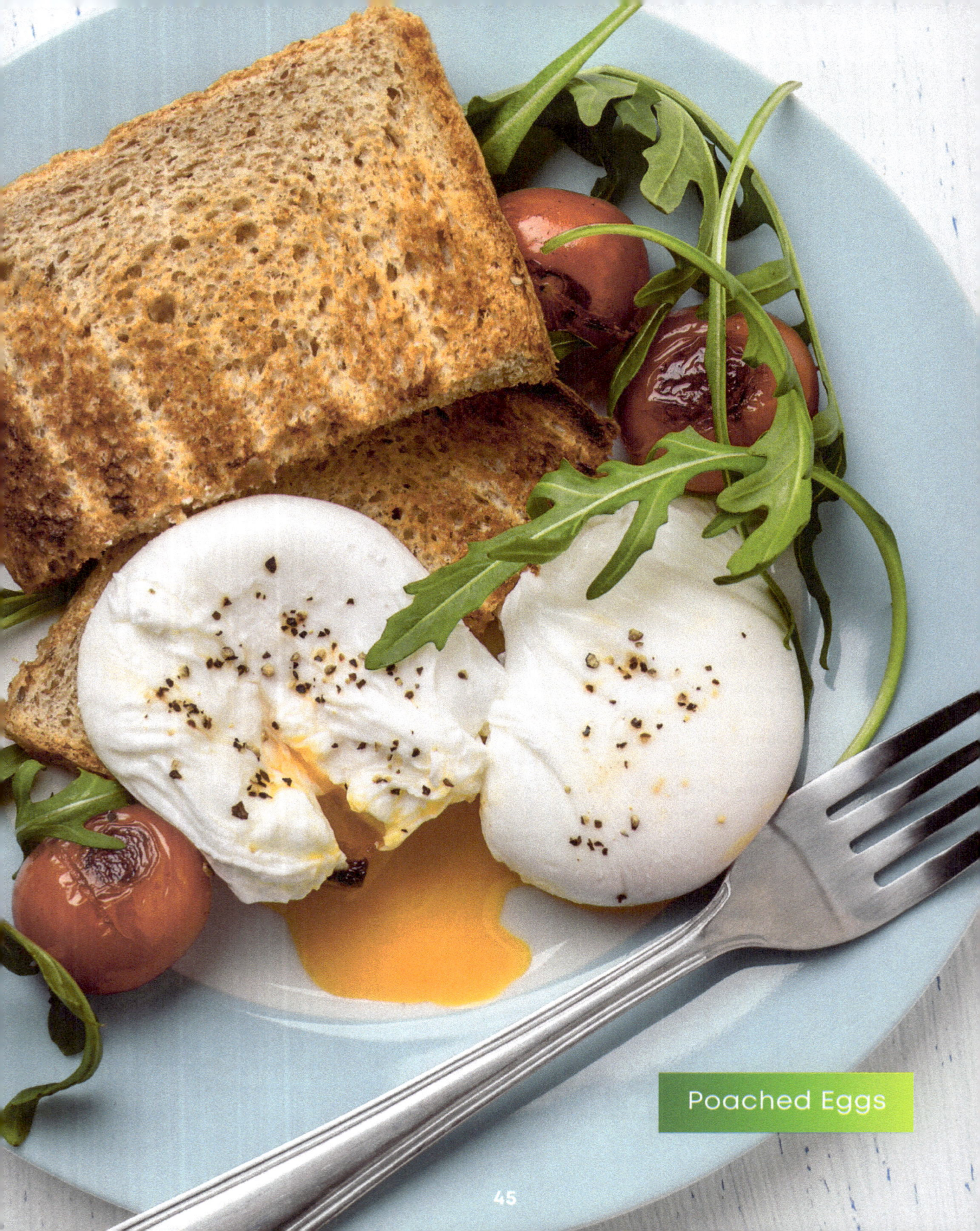
Poached Eggs

How to Poach an Egg
You need to learn how to do this. I promise it's easy!

SERVINGS: 2

INGREDIENTS

Water
Salt to season the water
FRESH eggs kept in the fridge until the very last minute
Vinegar is optional

METHOD

If you have only ever had disasters poaching, it was NOT YOUR FAULT.
It was simply an old egg so forgive yourself and try again.
Keep the eggs in the fridge until the very last minute, the colder the egg the better your 'luck' will be. I don't like the taste of vinegar so I don't add it. But you can add 10% vinegar to the water if you can handle the taste.

Grab a frying pan (you can use a saucepan, but a frying pan is easier to retrieve with the slotted spoon later). Grease the base of the frying pan with cooking spray or a little oil, preventing any accidents and sticking later. Fill the frying pan with hot water, enough to cover the height of the eggs. Season the water with about a teaspoon of salt.
Place the pan over a medium heat, the water should be at a gentle simmer not a boil.
Boiling water will agitate your eggs and break them up unnecessarily.
When the water is gently simmering, crack the eggs (as many as you need) carefully into the water. It's best to drop them into the water as low as you can manage.

Get your slotted spoon ready and keep the water simmering gently.

DO NOT LET THE WATER BOIL!

You might have to adjust as you go. You can see when the eggs are starting to set. For your first few times you can use the slotted spoon to check how cooked your egg is. If it is ready, take it out using the spoon and then drain it on some paper towel, just to drain the water. Getting rid of the water now will prevent soggy toast.
If the egg is 'wisping' in the water *(spreading out tendrils like a wisp of smoke)*, and if it looks like it may be falling apart, it may just be that the egg is old and that the egg white is old and thin. You can simply 'cut' this wispy egg off with the side of your spoon and they will look gorgeous again.
Practice makes perfect, and you will get better and better the more you make these.
Remember, you can add 10% of vinegar to help 'set' the eggs but it does dramatically change the flavour in my opinion.
Happy Poaching.

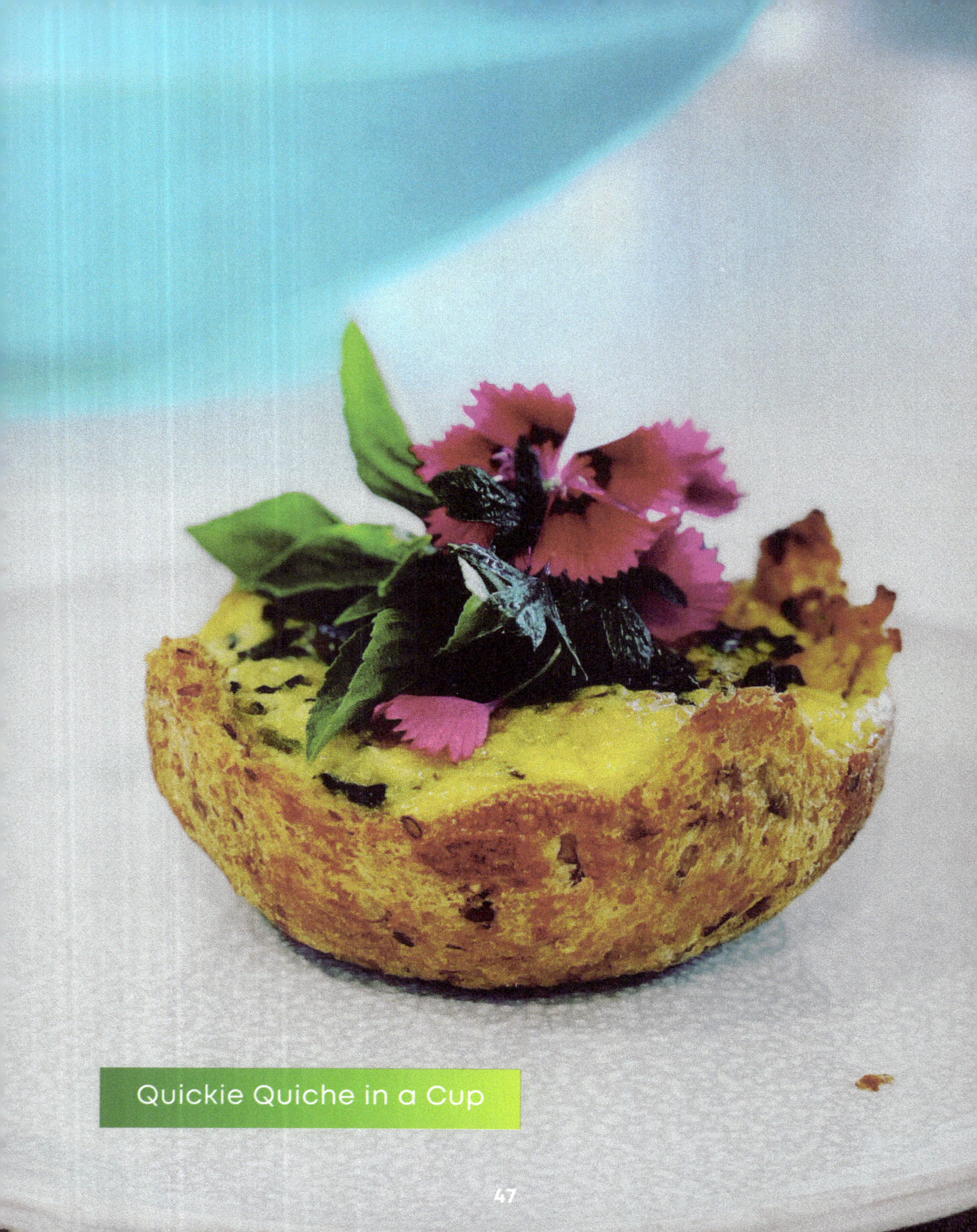

Quickie Quiche in a Cup

Quickie Quiche in a Cup

SERVINGS: 2

INGREDIENTS

2 slices of bread, buttered and crusts removed (low carb is perfect)
2 tablespoons cooked, chopped or diced bacon
OR prosciutto/pancetta OR speck OR chorizo sausage OR mushrooms
(you choose, this is perfect for leftovers)
2 tablespoons chopped onions
OR spinach OR spring onion OR zucchini OR tomato
3-4 fresh free-range eggs
1 pinch of pepper to season
1 tablespoon grated cheddar
Pecorino or parmesan (optional)

METHOD

**I absolutely make this all the time.
It's that quick, tasty fix that you just need some mornings... or even for a lunch!**

Grease the two heat-proof tea cups or ramekins, or a metal pie dish.
Take your buttered, crustless bread and push each one into the cup or ramekin.
Use your fingertips to press & mound the bread to the cup - it will be a very thin 'fake' pastry.

Now add your choice of fillings - you can literally add anything you like, but leave a little space for the egg mixture.

Beat the eggs and seasoning by whisking lightly with a fork.
Pour this egg mixture over the fillings and then top with the cheese.
Bake in a preheated oven at 180C for about 15 minutes, or until the egg is cooked.
You can also do this in your air fryer.

The bread will go nice and crispy.

So easy. Enjoy!

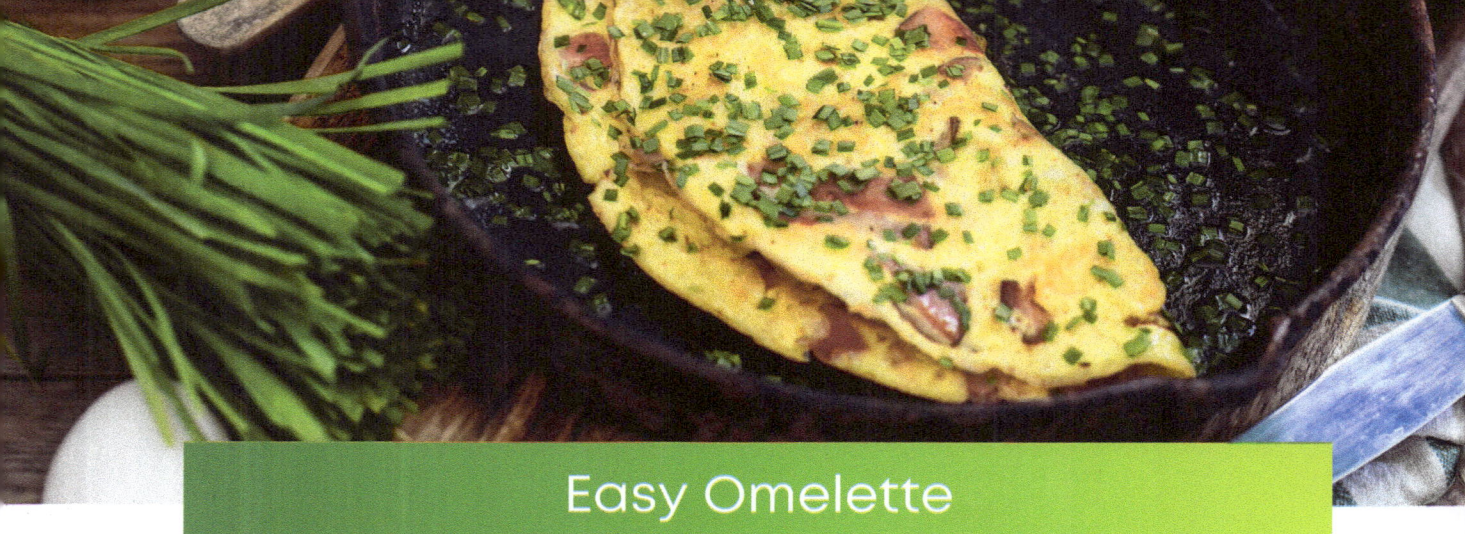

Easy Omelette

SERVINGS: 2-4

INGREDIENTS

OMLETTE	FILLINGS
1 teaspoon butter	2-4 tablespoons of the filling of your choice; chopped ham, spinach, bacon, mushrooms, onions, capsicum or cheese
2 eggs	
1 tablespoon finely chopped herbs of your choice	
1 tablespoon water	
1 pinch salt	
1 pinch pepper	

METHOD

To be honest... a great omelette is all about the pan. Go buy one if you have to.

You need a clean, non-stick pan or a stainless steel pan that is totally smooth. My preference is a non-stick.

Grease with a vegetable oil like sunflower or rice bran but NOT olive oil. Olive oil makes everything stick! Heat the pan gently with the butter. Place the eggs, herbs, seasoning and water into a bowl and beat to form a smooth batter.

When the butter is sizzling gently, pour the entire egg mixture into the pan. Get a plastic egg lift and start gently scraping the egg mix from the edge of the pan to the centre of the pan, as it sets. Do this about 4-6 times and then add the filling.

Now let the egg cook and form a brown crust, ensuring it is not sticking. If it has stuck, spray or grease more next time! Using your egg-lift, tilt the pan, and fold the omelette in half using the egg-lift to help. Slide it onto a plate and serve!

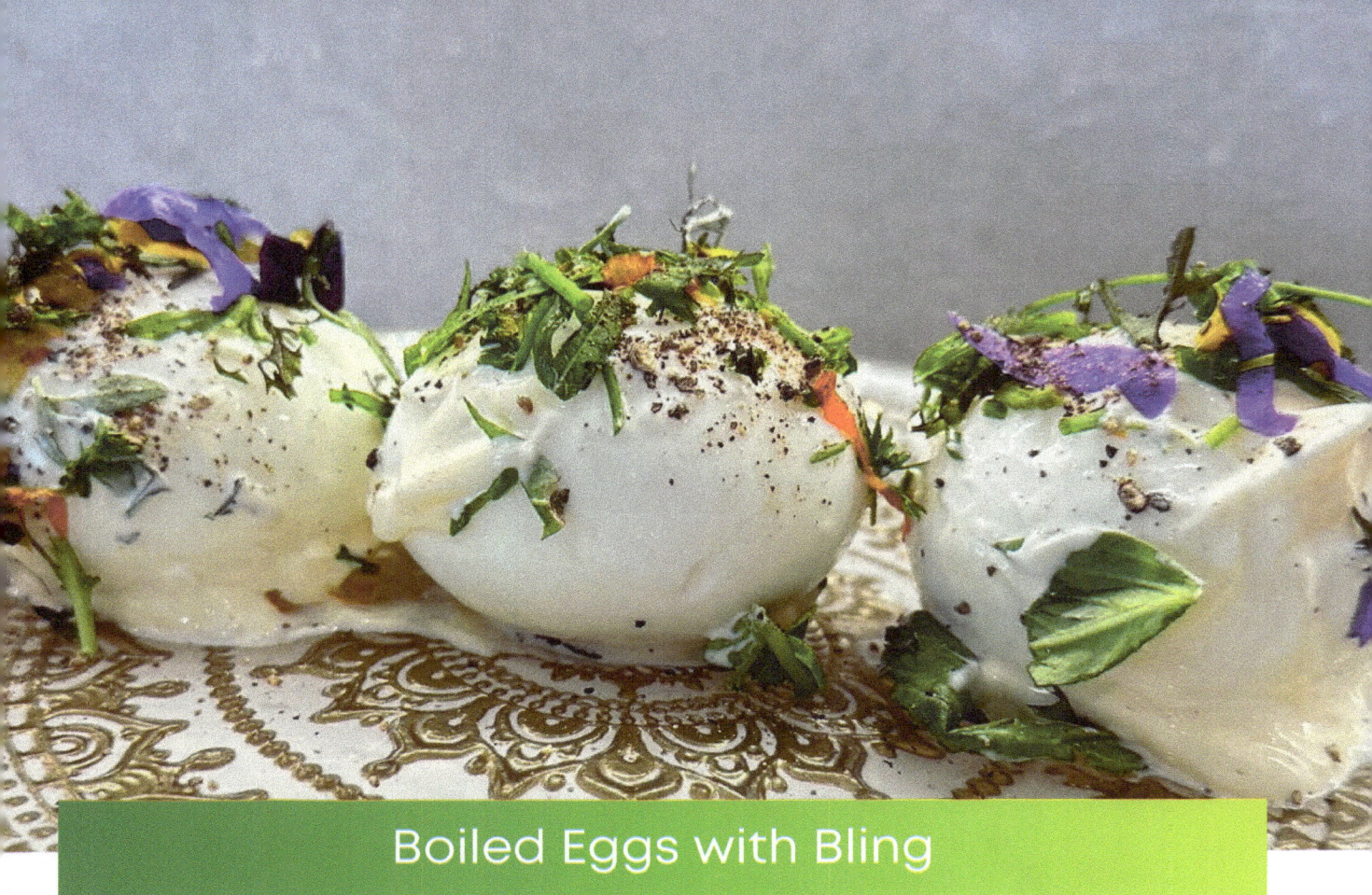

Boiled Eggs with Bling

SERVINGS: 1

INGREDIENTS

2 boiled eggs

GARNISH

2-4 tablespoons of green goodness of your choice
like chopped parsley, dill, chives, basil or sprouts
2 tablespoons of mayo or plain yogurt thinned with about 1 tablespoon water

METHOD

Boiled eggs can be pretty boring, but they are a valuable snack and an excellent source of protein for you.
They are also perfect to take to work as snacks, so we need to know how to pimp them up.

I boil my eggs, and then dress them with a little mayo thinned down with water to make a drizzling consistency, then add chopped herbs like basil or dill and lots of black pepper to make them sexy!

Enjoy!

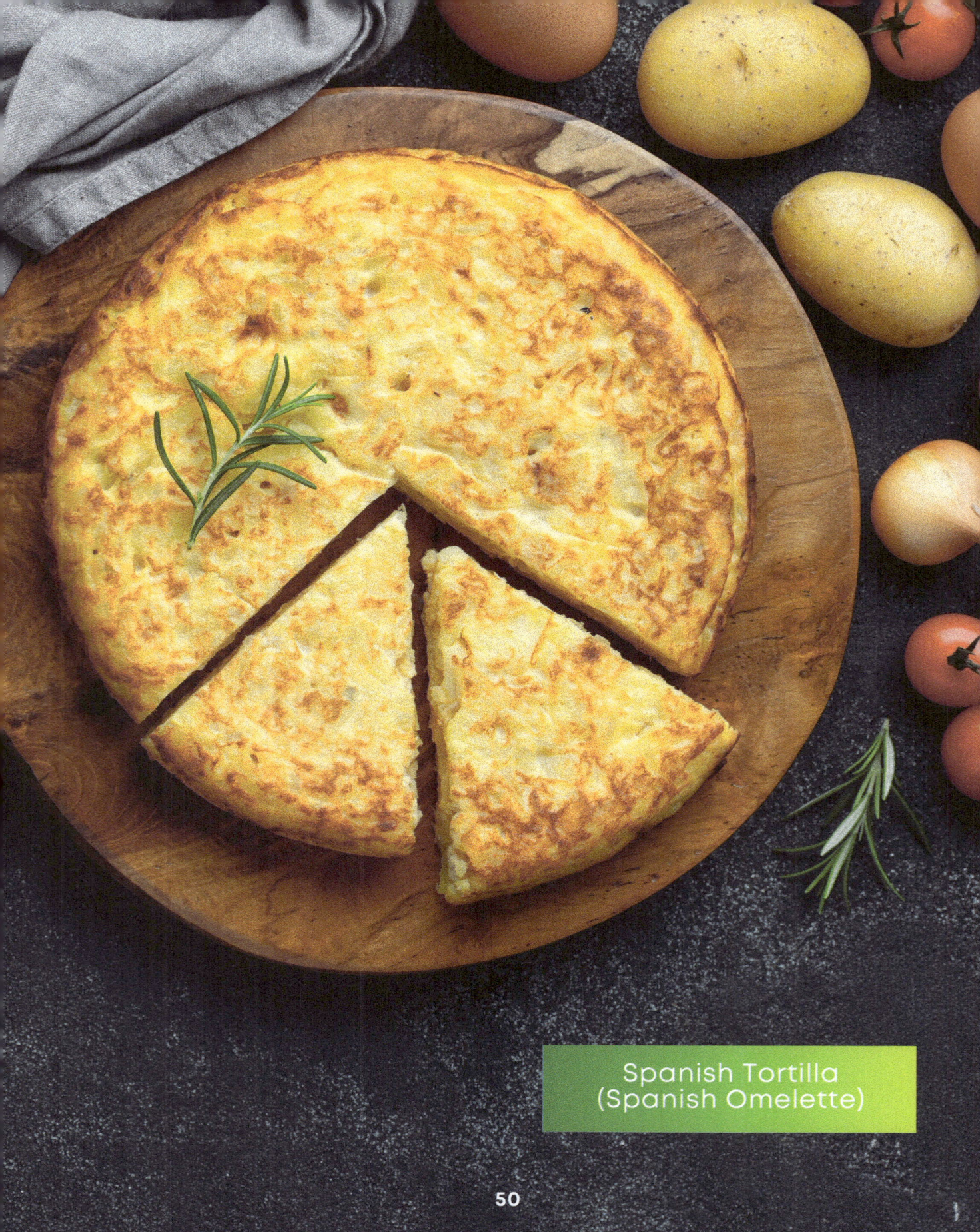

Spanish Tortilla (Spanish Omelette)

Spanish Tortilla

SERVINGS: 1

INGREDIENTS

1 small cooked and cooled potato, sliced thickly
1 egg beaten with 100ml milk or cream *or half-and-half*
3ml smoked paprika
1 tablespoon chopped parsley, chives, basil or sage… you choose!
1 small onion finely chopped
1 tablespoon chorizo, bacon, speck or mushrooms finely chopped

METHOD 1

Grease and heat a small non-stick frying pan with canola oil until it is swearword hot.
Add the chorizo or the alternative you are using, and allow to brown and the fat to render and then add the onion, chopped herbs and paprika.
Reduce heat and stir until onions are cooked and fragrant.

Now remove from the heat and layer your cooked potato over this delicious and very fragrant Spanish gravel. Mix the egg with the cream and/or milk and beat until smooth, season to taste with salt and pepper.
Pour over the potato and gravel, then bake in a hot oven (200C) for 8-12 minutes until the egg is set. Garnish, cut into triangles and serve as tapas with your other dishes!

So delicious, quick and healthy.

METHOD 2

You can use three whole eggs, unbeaten, cracked over this gravel as an alternative - makes a delicious breakfast dish. Omit the milk mentioned in the ingredients for this version.

Heat and grease the frying pan well, you DO NOT want to underdo the oiling and then all your ingredients stick. Place the diced bacon or its alternatives in the pan and let the meat or mushrooms go crisp and brown and flavoursome.

Now spread it evenly around the pan. Crack the eggs over this deliciousness and then turn the heat to medium, put the lid on the pan and let those eggs cook through to the doneness you like; soft, medium or hard.

Season with pepper, oil, and it's ready to serve!

Salads

Mix it Up!

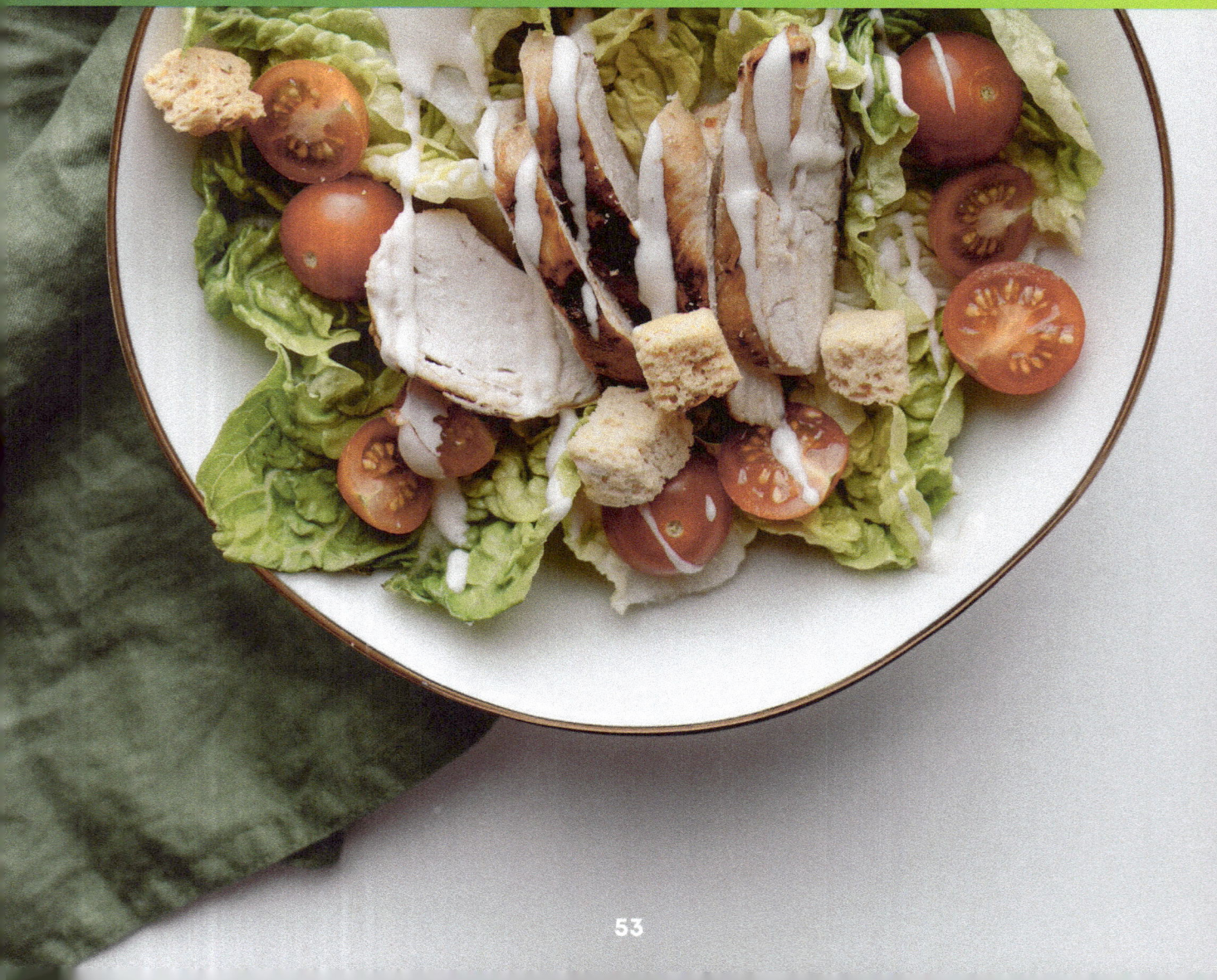

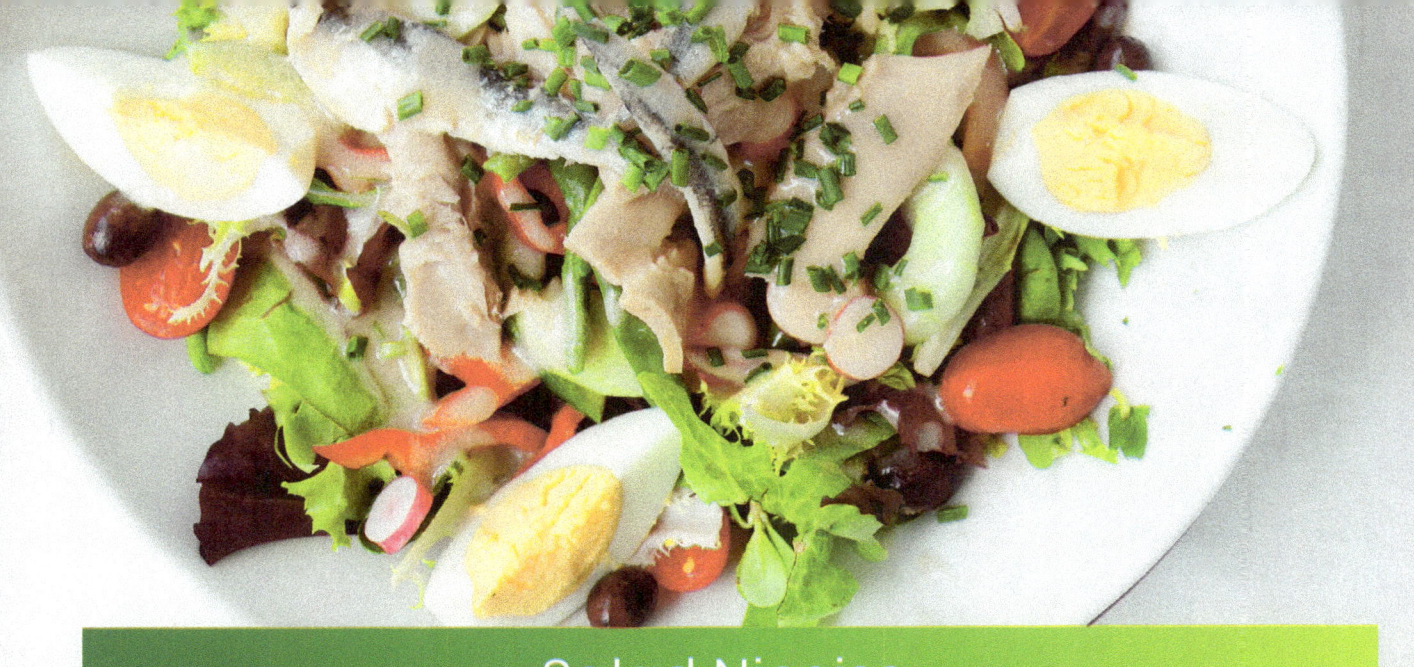

Salad Niçoise

SERVINGS: 1

INGREDIENTS

SALAD

6-8 baby green beans, trimmed
80g tuna flakes or chunks, drained
6-8 cherry tomatoes, halved
6-8 olives
1/2 baby cos lettuce heart, leaves separated, washed
1 hard-boiled egg, halved
3 anchovy fillets in oil, drained, halved lengthways (*optional*)

NICOISE DRESSING

3 tablespoons Extra Virgin Olive Oil
1 tablespoon Red Wine Vinegar
1 teaspoon Dijon mustard
Salt and pepper to season

METHOD

Salad Nicoise is an oldie but a goodie.

It has an amazing depth of flavour and personality and is a very respectable dinner party addition. ESPECIALLY if you use freshly seared fresh tuna instead of tinned.

But this one is an everyday adaptation so use that tin with pride.
Simply start by arranging the leaves in a sexy salad bowl, and top it with all the delicious beans, tuna, tomatoes, olives, egg and anchovies.

The dressing is just mixed together and then drizzled before serving.

Enjoy!

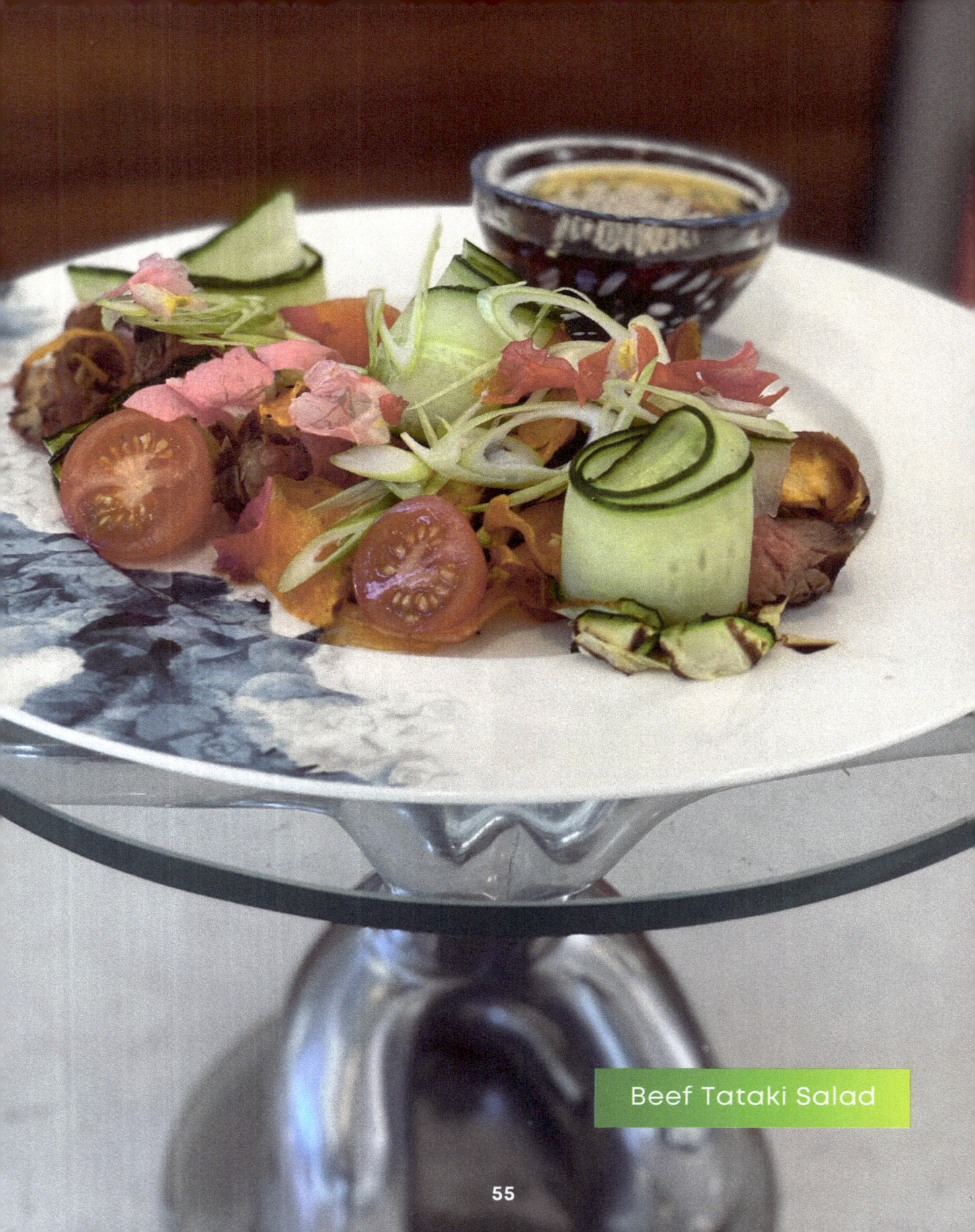
Beef Tataki Salad

Beef Tataki Salad

SERVINGS: 1

INGREDIENTS

SALAD

80-100g beef fillet or rump, salted and chargrilled *to rare or medium-rare as you prefer. You can do a whole beef fillet/tenderloin OR larger cut of rump like this if you are cooking for many)*
1 tablespoon teriyaki or oyster sauce
1/2 cup halved cherry tomatoes
1/2 cup cucumber ribbons or cubed
1/2 zucchini, cut into ribbons or diced
3 spring onions, finely chopped
1 teaspoon toasted sesame seeds to garnish

SAUCE

2 tablespoons mirin
2 tablespoons cooking wine/rice wine
2 tablespoons soy sauce
1 clove garlic crushed or grated
1 teaspoon grated ginger

METHOD

Mix your sauce ingredients together and place in a large bowl. Set aside.
Grease and heat a frying pan with some vegetable oil.
Season your steak with salt and pepper; a room temp steak will be the best!

Once the pan is swearword hot, place the steak in the pan and let it seal for about 2 minutes on the first side. Only when you have the perfect crust should you turn it over and do the other side.
With all steaks, but especially thin ones, the pan should be swearword hot. A thin steak cooked in a cold pan will be a grey disaster.

Once the steak is sealed and brown and gorgeous on both sides, remove it from the pan and allow it to rest in the bowl with the sauce ingredients. You can cook the steak further to how you like it of course. Resting the steak in the sauce allows it to not only cool quicker but also to grab all that lovely flavour.

Allow to cool completely on the bench, or put in the fridge and use over the next few days.

Once cool, remove from the sauce.
Carve into thin slices and assemble on a plate with the rest of the salad and vegetable ingredients.
Dress with some of the remaining sauce and toasted sesame seeds.

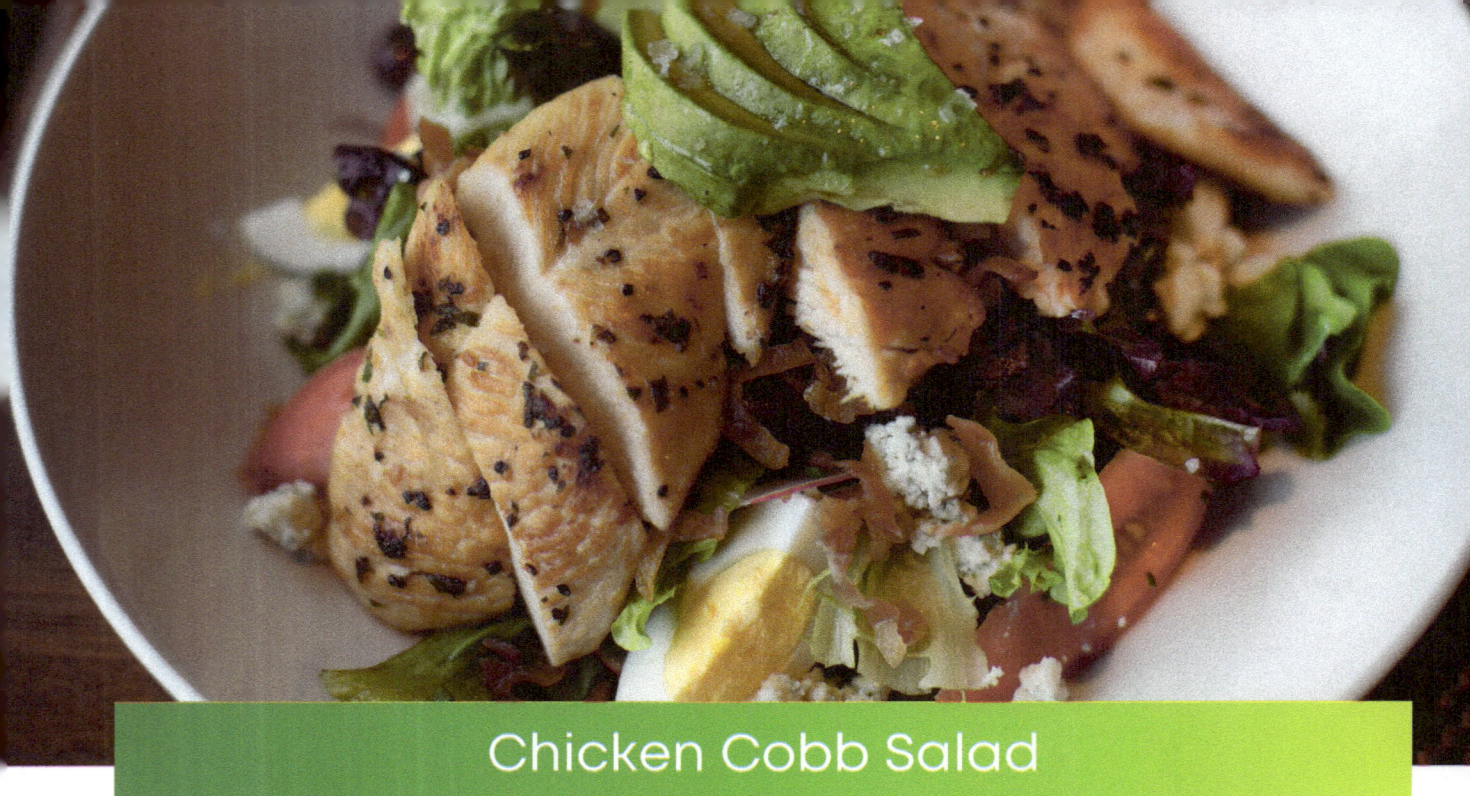

Chicken Cobb Salad

SERVINGS: 1

INGREDIENTS

SALAD
- 80-100g cooked shredded chicken
- 1 soft-boiled egg, halved
- 1/2 cup halved cherry tomatoes
- 1/2 avocado, diced or sliced
- 1/2 red onion finely sliced or diced
- 1/2 head romaine, iceberg or cos lettuce
- 2 slices streaky bacon, cooked and diced

DRESSING
- 1 tablespoon blue cheese
- 1 tablespoon mayo or fat free yogurt
- 2 tablespoons water
- All mixed to a paste

METHOD

Make this for yourself or make it for the family!

Place the lettuce leaves in a bowl and add the chopped tomatoes and onions over the leaves.

Top with the shredded chicken, avo and bacon and then dress with the super simple dressing.

This salad is so delicious I would even serve it as a dinner party main during the summer months.

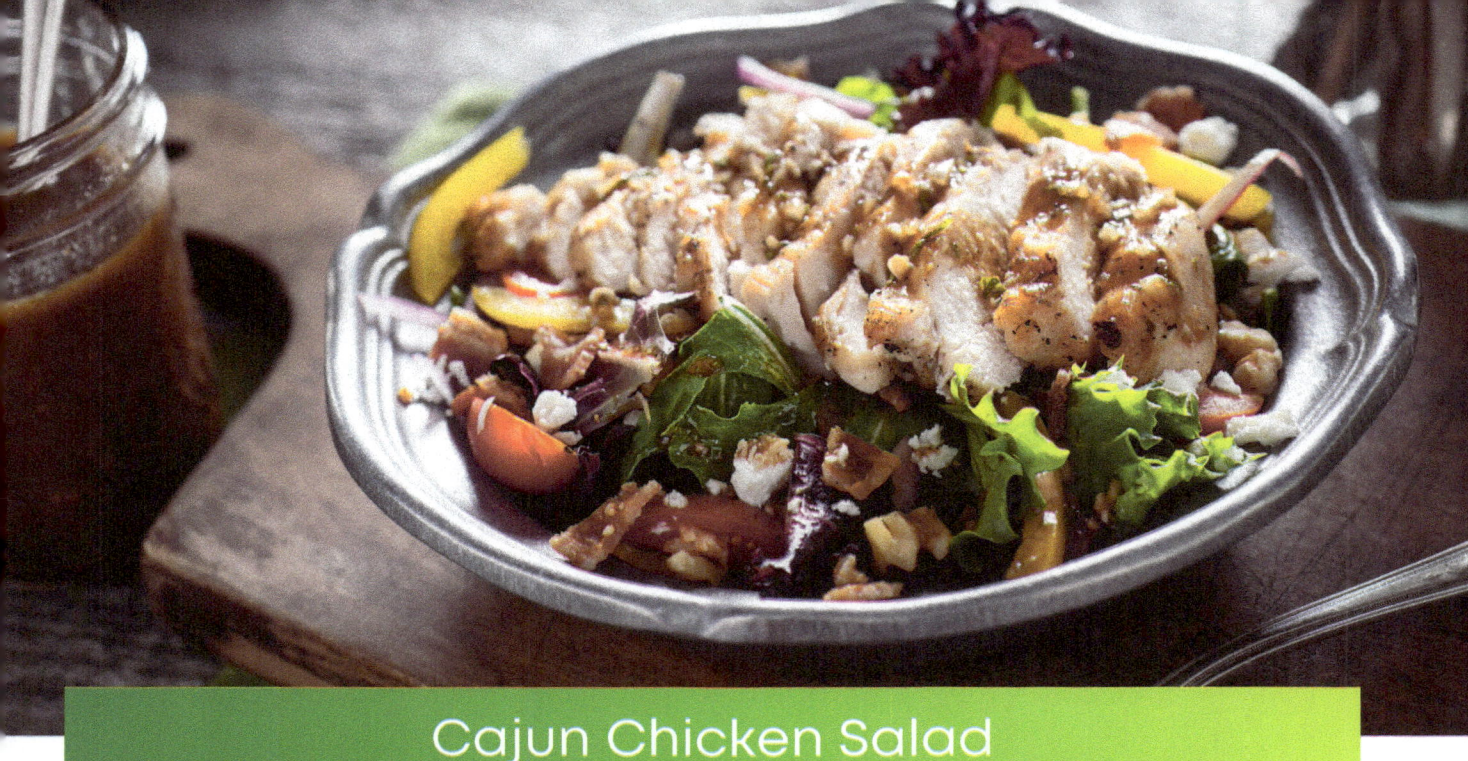

Cajun Chicken Salad

SERVINGS: 1

INGREDIENTS

SALAD

80-100g cooked, shredded chicken
1/2 head romaine, iceberg or cos lettuce
1/2 cup halved cherry tomatoes
1/2 cup cooked or grilled corn
1/2 red onion finely sliced or diced
1/2 avocado diced or sliced
1/2 sliced red or green capsicum/pepper
2 slices streaky bacon cooked and diced

DRESSING

1 tablespoon mayo OR fat free plain yogurt
1/4 teaspoon Cajun seasoning
2 tablespoons water
All mixed to a paste

METHOD

Perfect to use up leftover chicken OR beef, or pimp up a tin of chickpeas if you prefer.

Start by placing the lettuce leaves, corn, chopped tomatoes and onions on a plate or bowl.

Top with the shredded chicken, avocado, capsicum/pepper and bacon and then dress with the super simple dressing.

I love this salad and the quick and easy dressing. So versatile.

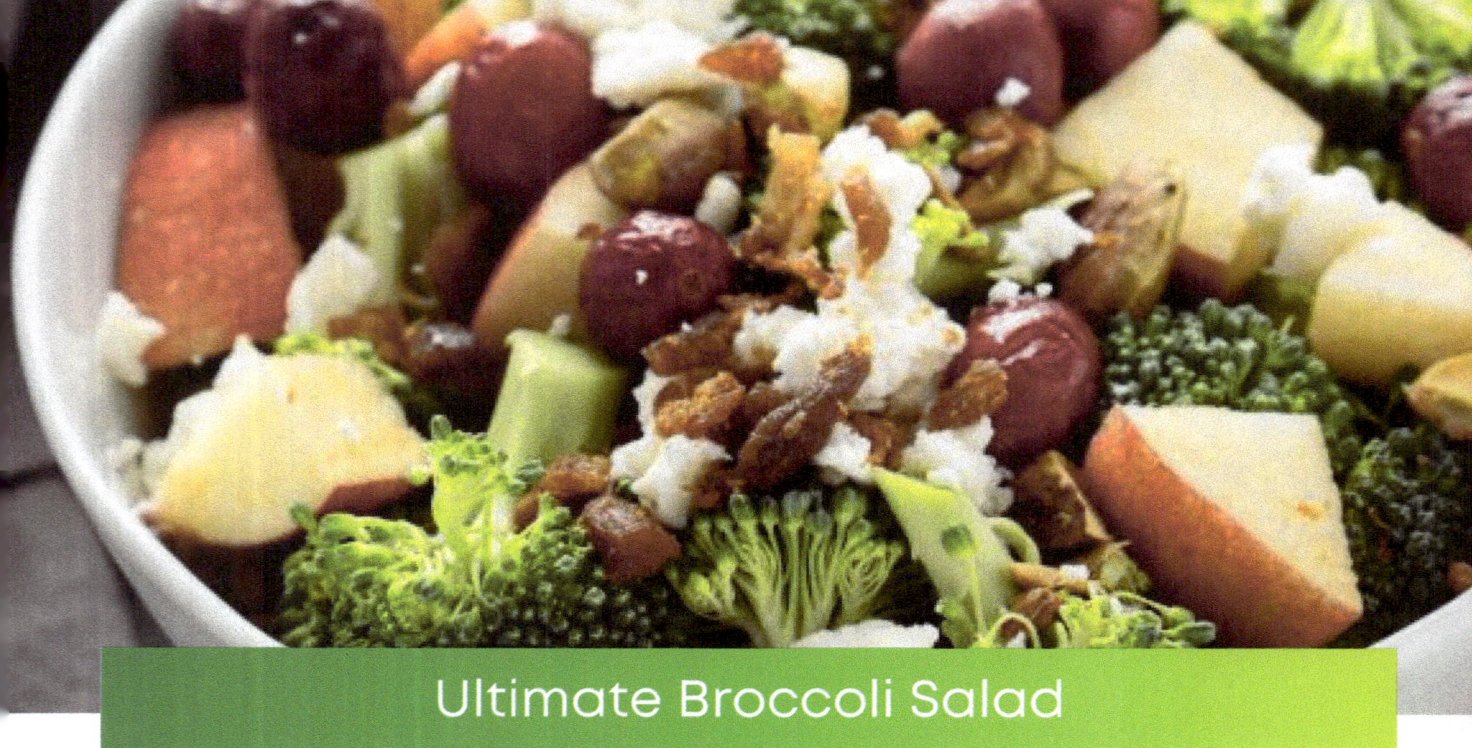

Ultimate Broccoli Salad

SERVINGS: 2-4

INGREDIENTS

SALAD

Mix and match with what you prefer
1 head broccoli, chopped into a 'rice' using a sharp knife
Or by blending in the food processor
2-3 rashers streaky bacon cooked until crisp and then chopped up finely or use 1 cup shredded chicken or even a tin of tuna

1 red onion finely diced
1 cup finely chopped cabbage, carrots or brussels sprouts
1 tablespoon chopped almonds or pine nuts

DRESSING

1 teaspoon grainy or Dijon mustard
4 tablespoons plain Greek or fat-free yogurt

METHOD

Want a salad that is healthy AND delicious?
I love this salad, I make it so often and in so many different ways, even my fussy kids love it.

I often have it as my main or I'll serve it as a side at a dinner party.

The yogurt and mustard dressing keep this salad light and nutritious.
You can prepare all the veggies in advance and then dress just before you serve or else it will keep for a day or two in the fridge. Simply toss all the ingredients into a bowl, dress and enjoy!

Changing the protein will make sure you enjoy this salad many times.

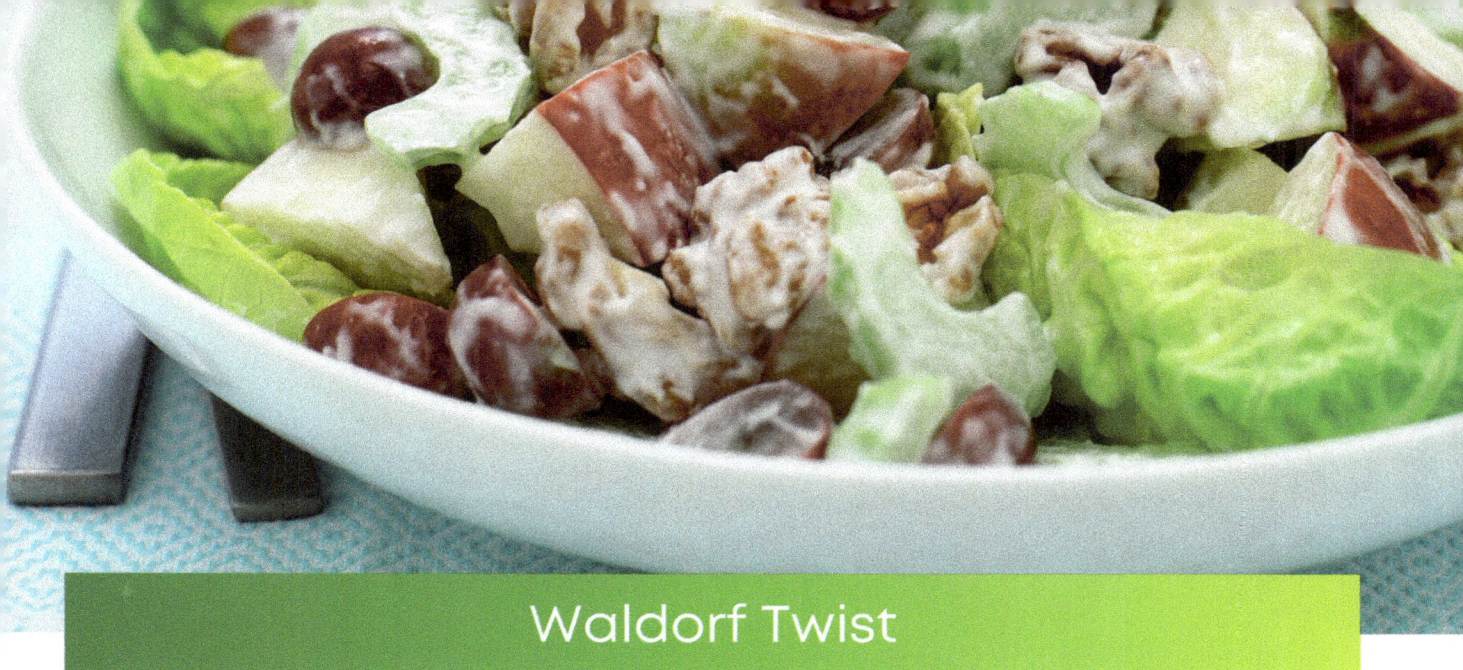

Waldorf Twist

SERVINGS: 1

INGREDIENTS

SALAD

- 80-100g cooked shredded chicken
- 1/2 cup chopped celery
- 1/2 apple, cored and diced
- 1 tablespoon diced brie or camembert (optional)
- 1 tablespoon diced walnuts
- *(please make sure they are fresh and not stale!)*
- 1/2 head romaine, iceberg or cos lettuce
- 2 slices streaky bacon, cooked and diced
- 1 teaspoon raisins or cranberries

DRESSING

- 1 tablespoon mayo
- 1/2 teaspoon mustard
- 2 tablespoons water mixed to a paste

METHOD

A traditional Waldorf salad is fabulous, but why not try this more substantial version as a healthy main course option?

The crunch and sweetness of the apple, combined with the savoury cheese and chicken, along with the crunch of the nuts makes this a very pleasurable meal indeed.

Enjoy, and leave out what you don't like.

Simply build this salad on a plate starting with the leaves, and then topping with the remaining ingredients and then finally the dressing.

Yummy!

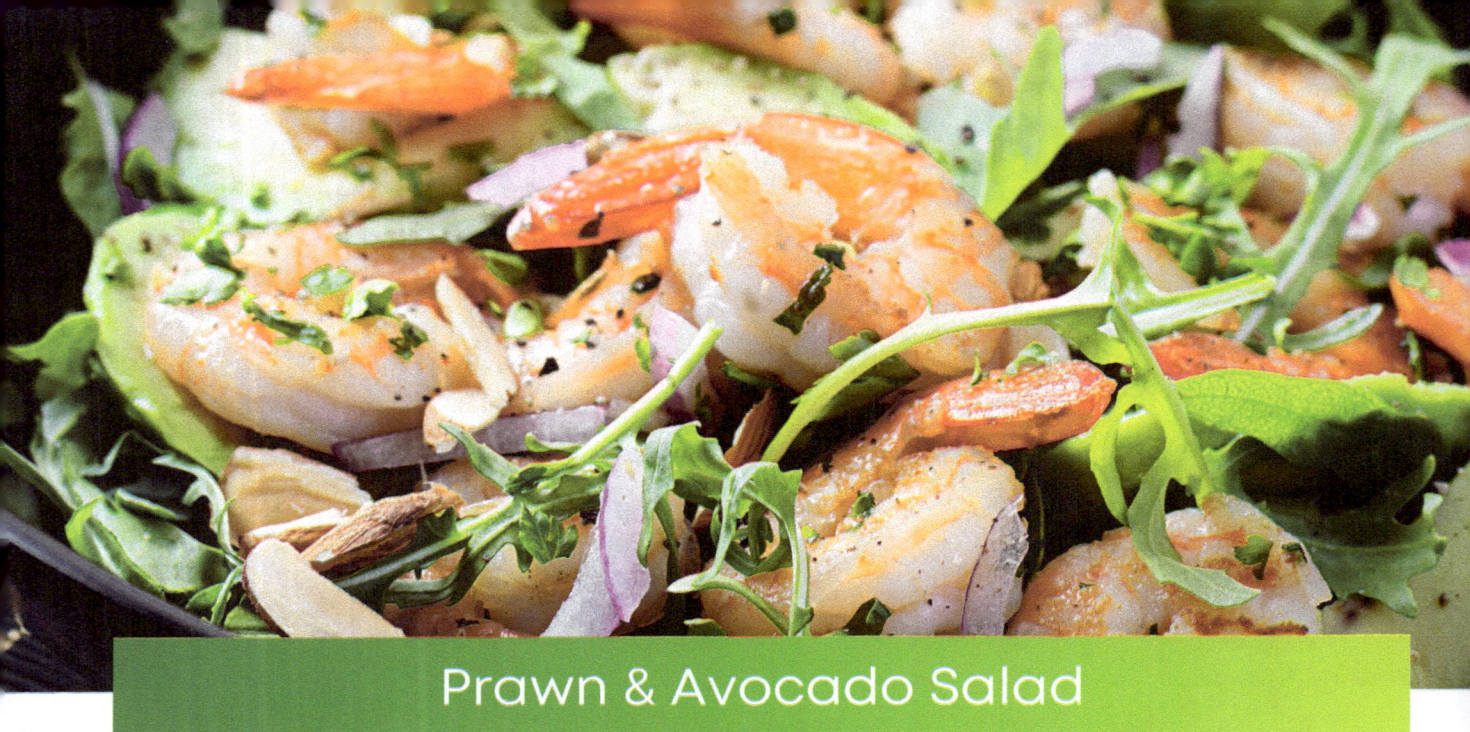

Prawn & Avocado Salad

SERVINGS: 2-3

INGREDIENTS

150-300g cooked and peeled prawns
2 avocados, diced
1 cup cherry tomatoes, halved
1/4 cup chopped red onion
1/4 cup chopped coriander/cilantro
1 jalapeño, finely chopped (optional, for some heat)
2 tablespoons lime juice
2 tablespoons olive oil
Salt and pepper to taste
Mixed salad greens for serving

METHOD

In a large bowl, combine the cooked prawns, diced avocados, cherry tomatoes, red onion, coriander/cilantro, and jalapeño (if using).

In a separate small bowl, whisk together the lime juice, olive oil, salt, and pepper to create the dressing. Drizzle the dressing over the shrimp and avocado mixture, and gently toss to coat everything evenly. Serve the prawn and avocado salad over a bed of mixed salad greens.
Such a lovely treat!

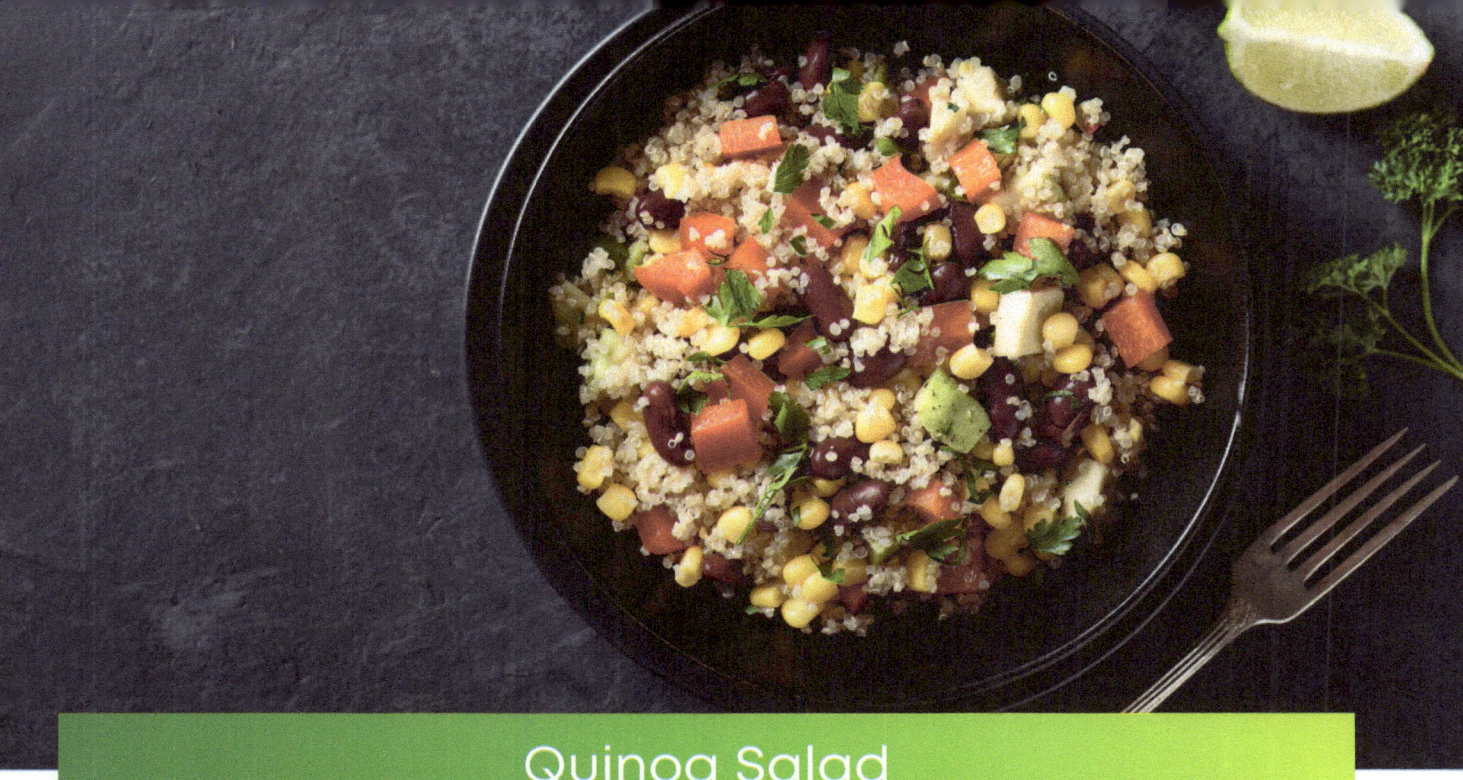

Quinoa Salad

SERVINGS: 2-3

INGREDIENTS

SALAD
1 cup quinoa, soaked as per package instructions
1/4 cup diced cucumber
1/4 cup corn kernels
1/4 sliced red onion
1/4 your choice protein (chicken/tuna/beef/tofu)
1/4 cup sliced tomato
1 cup spinach leaves or rocket
1 chili finely chopped
1/4 grated cheddar or use feta

DRESSING
1 tablespoon dairy cream
OR coconut cream OR mayo
1 tablespoon freshly chopped coriander or parsley
2 tablespoon extra virgin olive oil
1 tablespoon fresh lemon or lime juice
Salt and pepper to season

METHOD

For the dressing, simply combine the ingredients and stir together.
Mix and dress in a large bowl when ready to serve.

Serve into plates, season and enjoy.

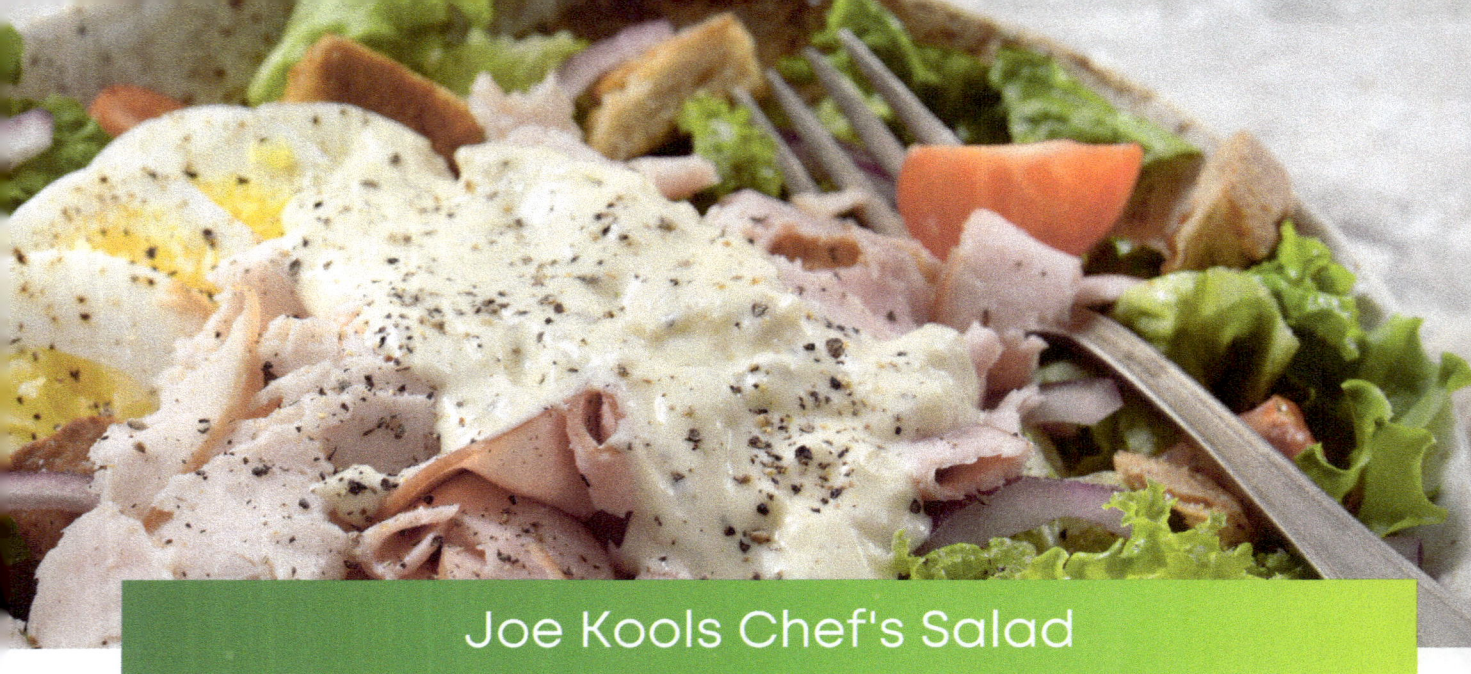

Joe Kools Chef's Salad

SERVINGS: 1

INGREDIENTS

SALAD
1/2 red onion, finely sliced or diced
1/2 head romaine, iceberg or cos lettuce
1/2 cup halved cherry tomatoes
1/2 sliced red or green capsicum/pepper
40g cooked shredded chicken
40g cooked shredded ham
20g grated cheddar cheese

DRESSING
1 tablespoon mayo
2 tablespoons water
mixed to a paste

METHOD

When I was studying we used to head to Joe Kools, our favourite pub on the beach on the Durban beachfront. This is my favourite salad of all time and is a very special memory indeed. It was on their menu for years and I often make it at home so I wanted to share it with you.

Place the lettuce leaves in a bowl and add the capsicum/pepper, chopped tomatoes and onions over the leaves.

Top with the shredded chicken, ham and cheese and then dress with the super simple dressing.

I love this salad and the quick and easy dressing. The memory of Joe Kools will live on through us!

Bowls & Stacks

Mix it Up!

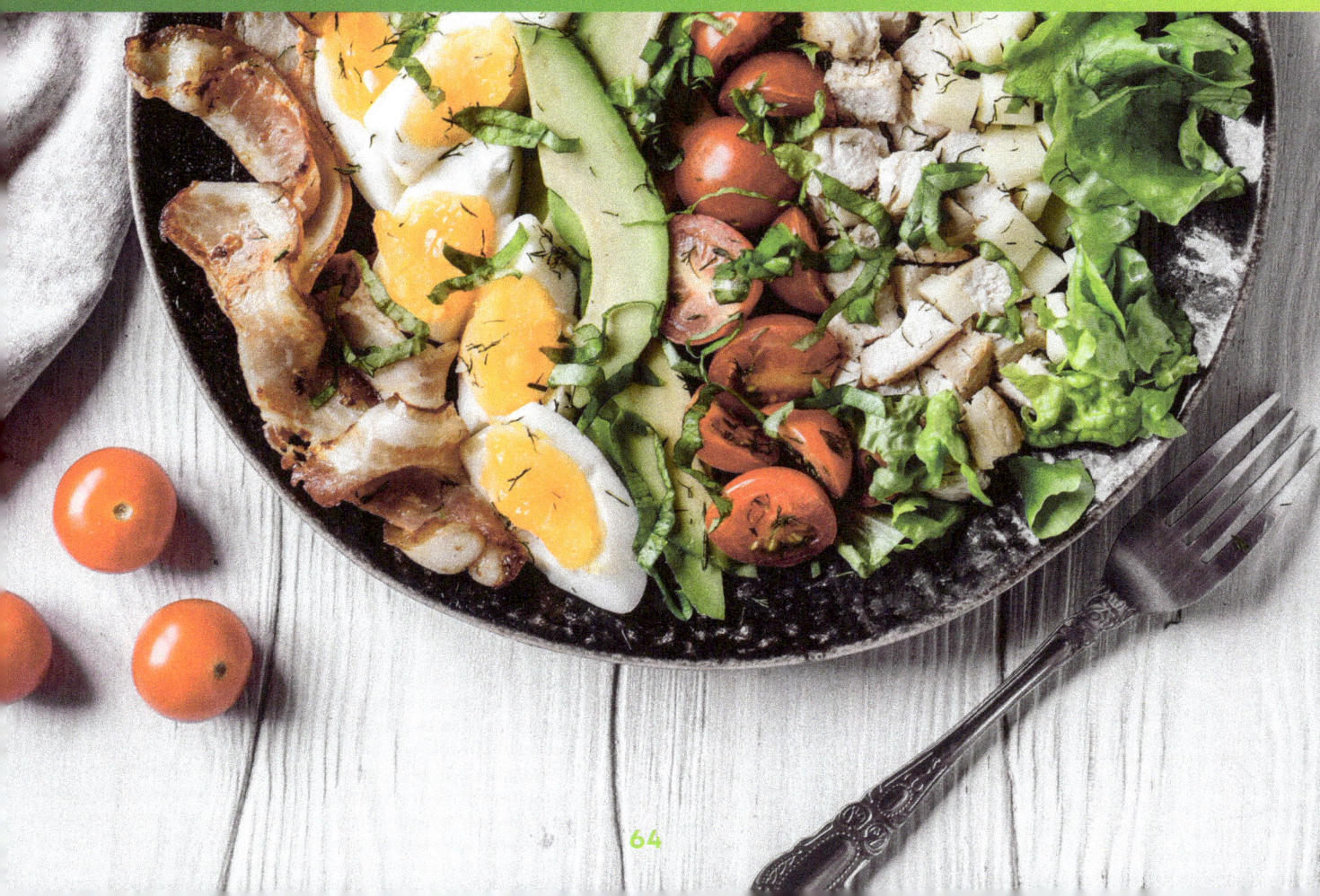

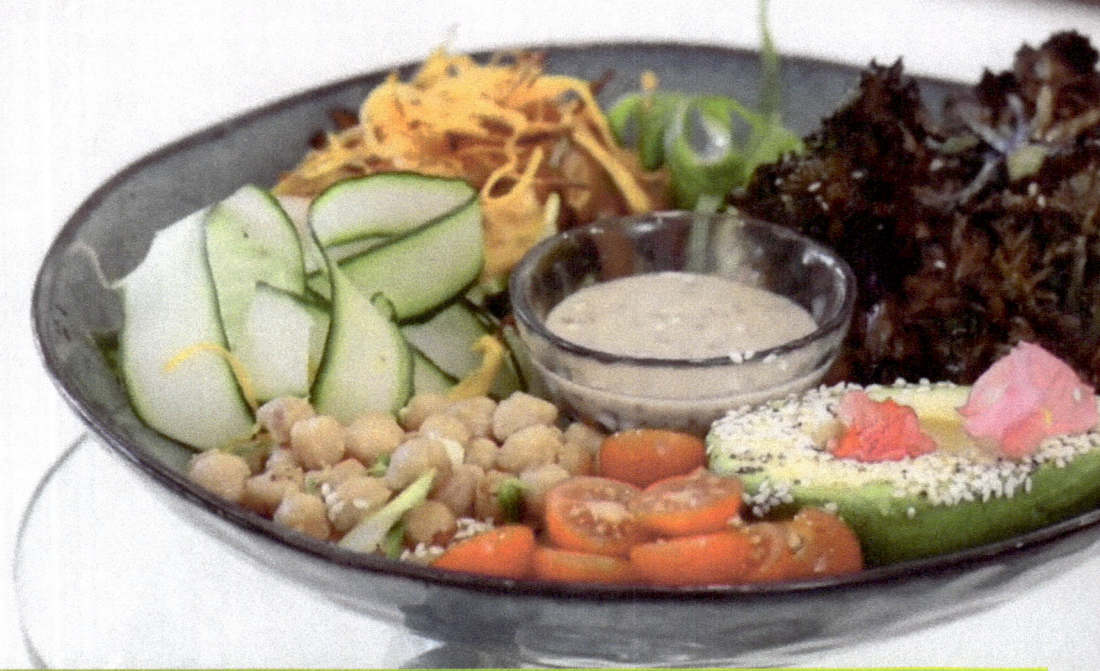

Miso Chick Pea Goodie Bowl

SERVINGS: 2

INGREDIENTS

SALAD

1 tin chickpeas, drained
1 tablespoon miso paste
1 cup finely sliced spinach
1 cup grated carrots
1 cup finely sliced cabbage or brussels sprouts
1/2 an avocado diced or fanned
Sesame seeds toasted for garnish

DRESSING

50ml kewpie mayo mixed with
50 ml water
and three drops sesame oil.

METHOD

Heat and grease a large frying pan. Add the drained chickpeas and the miso and simply heat through. You can either serve them hot or allow them to cool.

In a gorgeous bowl, arrange the miso chickpeas, avocado and veg around the salad dressing which has been placed in a small bowl.

It looks so pretty with all the gorgeous fresh ingredients arranged like this.
To eat, simply drizzle the dressing over the individual ingredients and then stir and enjoy.

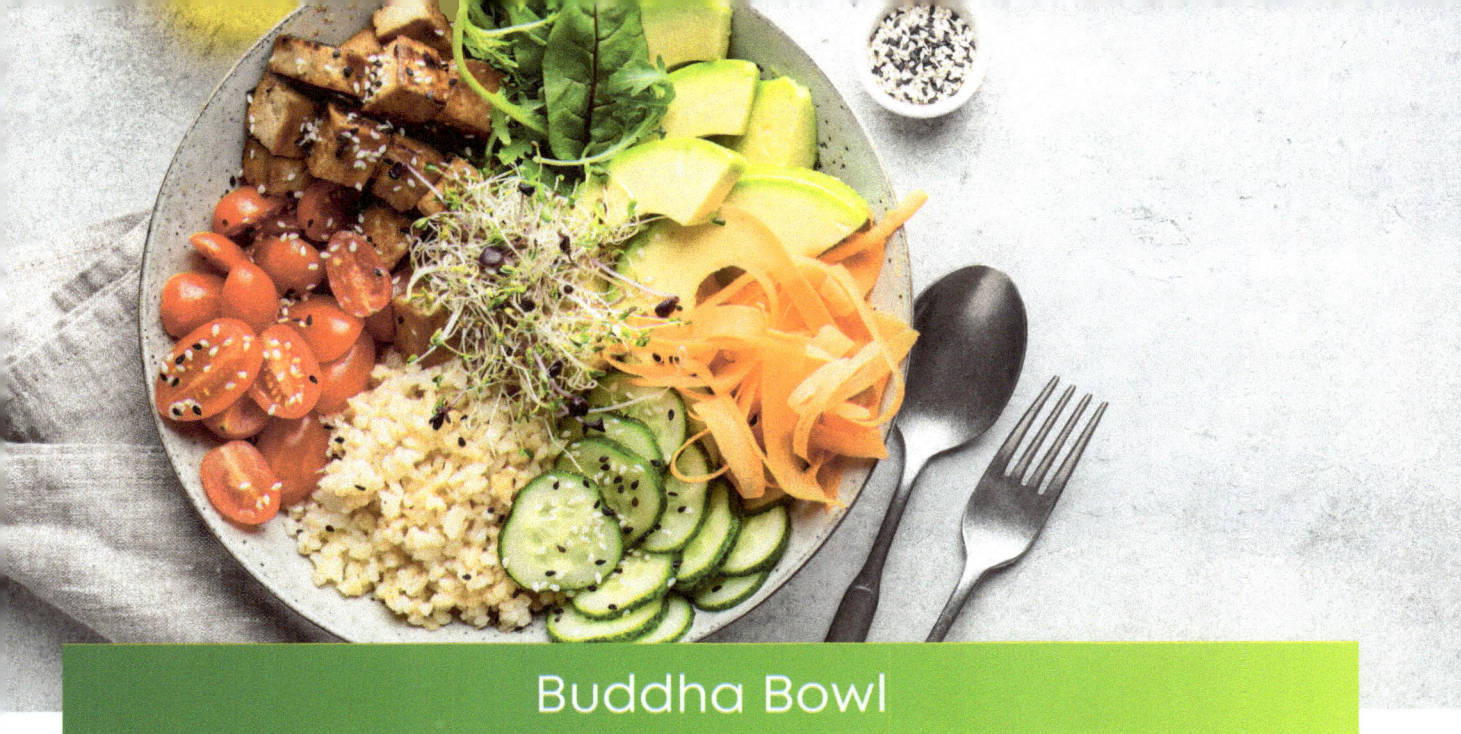

Buddha Bowl

SERVINGS: 2

INGREDIENTS

SALAD

1 cup diced cold chicken, tuna or beef
...*or anything you feel like*
1 cup diced or riced broccoli
1 cup finely diced spinach
1 cup grated carrots
1/2 cup halved cherry tomatoes
1 cup finely sliced cabbage or Brussels sprouts
Sesame seeds toasted for garnish

DRESSING

50ml mayo mixed with 50 ml water and big pinch crushed pepper, chopped chilli or chopped herbs

METHOD

A BUDDHA BOWL is a fantastic way to serve leftovers and lots of vegetables.

You can use any protein you like, and clean out the fridge and use all the veggies that need to be used.

I love how this colourful bowl looks so impressive, yet it's cheap and easy and delicious to make. Simply place all your ingredients in your bowl, add the dressing and enjoy.

Have fun, be creative, and you never have to have the same combination twice...unless you want to.

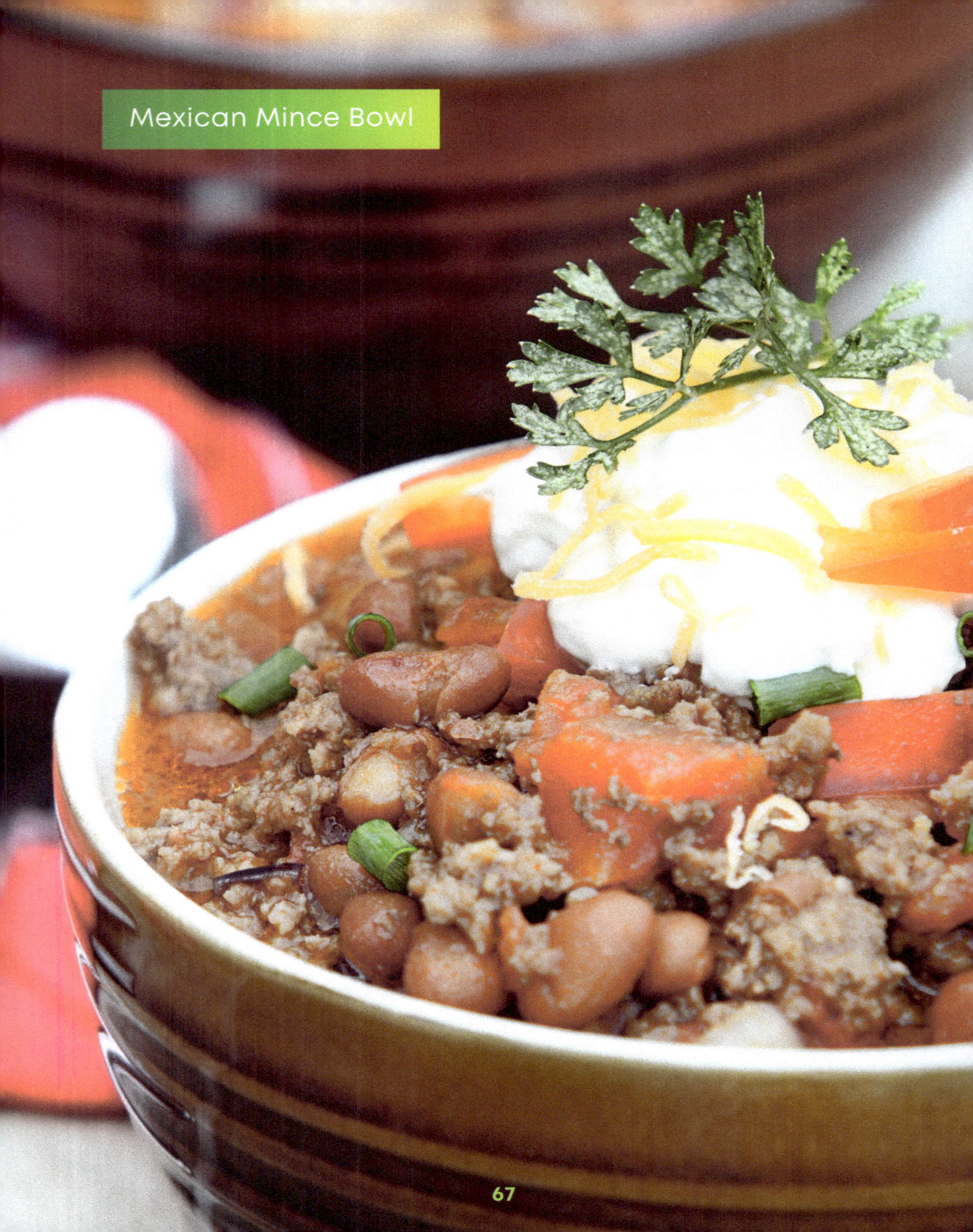

Mexican Mince Bowl

Mexican Mince Bowl

SERVINGS: 4-6

INGREDIENTS

SALAD
Canola or rice bran cooking spray
800g lean beef mince
1 large onion, finely diced
1 clove garlic, crushed (optional)
3 tablespoons Mexican Spice Mix
1 cup chopped tomatoes
1 vegetable or beef stock cube, crumbled to a powder
Salt & pepper to season
1 tin black beans

TOPPING
Sour Cream
1 avocado, chopped
1 bunch coriander/cilantro, chopped
1 chopped chilli
2 tablespoons crushed or bashed corn chips

METHOD

Grease a large pan with two squirts of cooking spray and heat until just about smoking hot. The mince MUST sizzle when it hits the pan.

Meanwhile, break up the mince in the packet or a bowl so it is loose and fluffy already. Put the mince into the pan…IT SHOULD SIZZLE nice and loud and sexy. DO NOT STIR, I know you are worried about this burning and you are also worried about lumps, but let the mince brown and seal on the first side you put down FIRST and let the pan heat up again and THEN you can stir ever so slightly just to get some more mince onto the base of the pan.

My favourite mince 'fluffer' is one of those cheap plastic-coated whisks you get at the supermarket that only have about 4 loops. If you don't have one of those, a strong plastic spoon or egg flip works well to help you break down the mince.

Once the mince is brown and fragrant and sexy ALL BY ITSELF, then and only then, do you add the finely chopped onion and garlic. There should be a good amount of fat rendered out of the mince during your amazing sizzling at a nice high heat.

You can stir as much as you like now by the way. That mince is SEALED off!

Now add the spices, stock powder and seasoning and stir through. Amazing colour isn't it?

Finally, add the chopped tomatoes. Turn down the heat and let that all cook through and then adjust your seasoning. This way of cooking will not only save you time, BUT it will add valuable flavour and vibrant personality to your otherwise boring mince.

I love to get creative with my mince and change the spices thus changing the flavour.

Serve in a bowl, topped with a dollop of sour cream, chopped avo, chopped coriander and chilli, and finally a lovely crunchy topping of crushed corn chips.

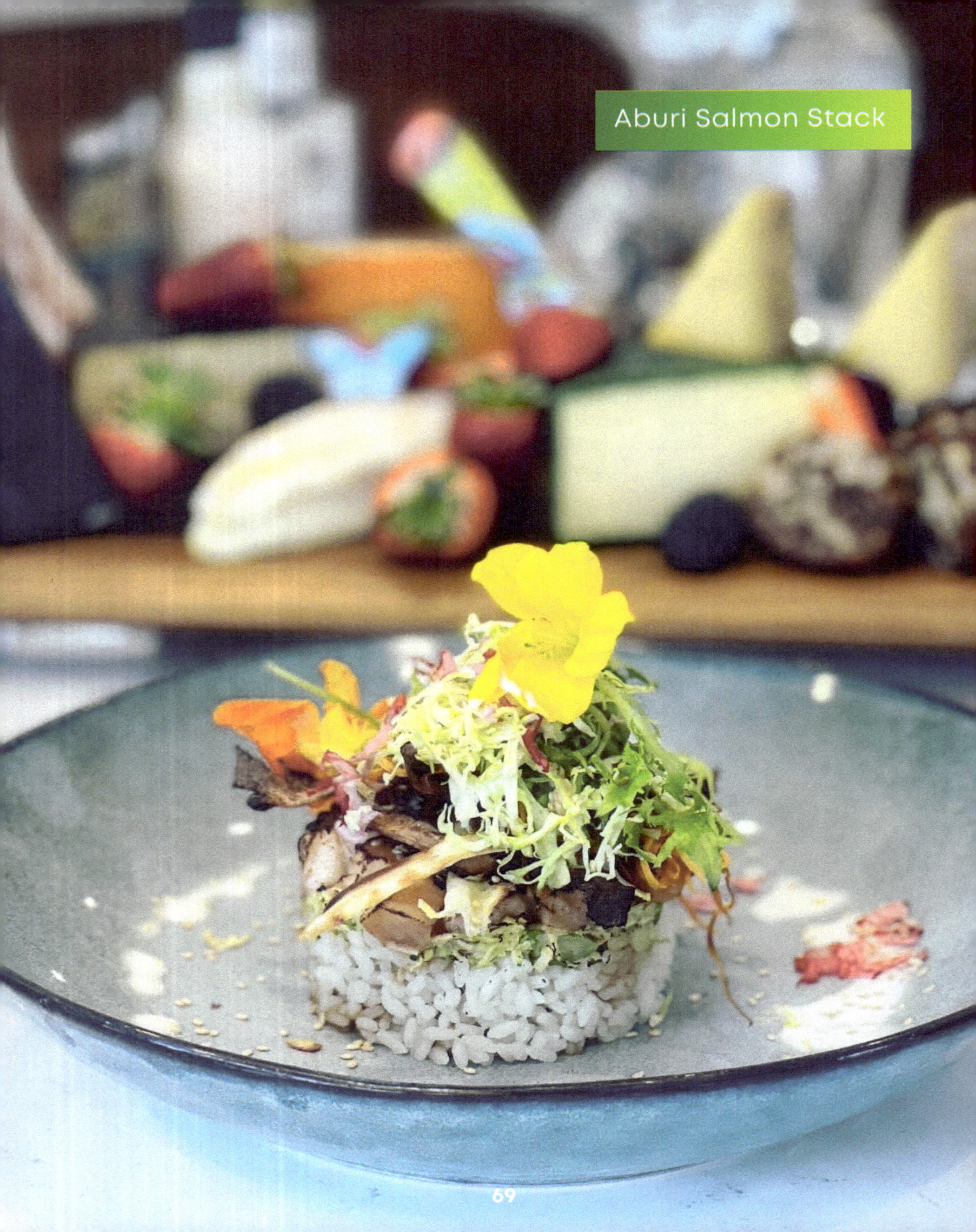

Aburi Salmon Stack

Aburi Salmon Stack

SERVINGS: 1

INGREDIENTS

80-100g raw salmon, finely chopped or sliced
1 tablespoon teriyaki or oyster sauce
1 cup broccoli chopped finely until it resembles rice
2-3 tablespoons prepared sushi rice or use cauliflower rice instead
50ml kewpie mayo mixed with 50 ml water and three drops sesame oil

METHOD

NOTE: Please don't be intimidated because this requires a blow torch.
A blow torch is easy and fun, but you can also pop this under the grill or cook in a frying pan, and get a similar result.

Dress the broccoli rice and sushi rice with the mayo, water and sesame oil and mix to form a lovely slaw.

Brush or mix the raw salmon in the teriyaki or oyster sauce and then 'scorch' with a blow torch until nicely cooked and browned on the edges OR pop under a pre-heated grill as close as you can get it to the element, until the salmon is cooked and browned.

So easy, and one of my favourite cheat ways to prepare fish into a sexy salad.

Once done, you can then assemble on a plate and serve.
I like to make a base of the raw slaw and then top it with the salmon.
I sometimes use a cheffy stacking ring to form the slaw into a neat tower, top it with the scorched salmon and serve!
I love these easy but delicious cheats!

"Laughter is brightest where food is best!"
— Irish Proverb

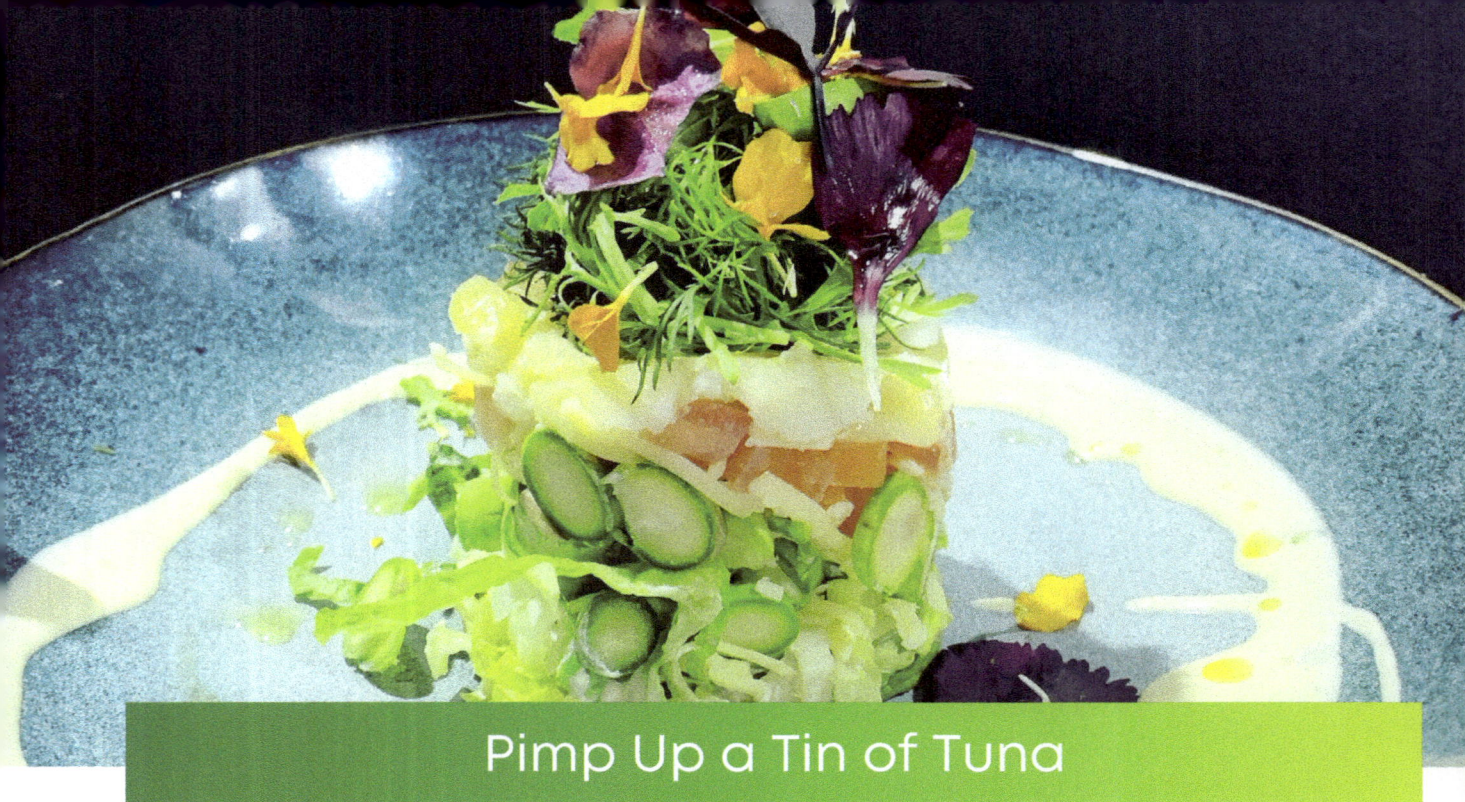

Pimp Up a Tin of Tuna

SERVINGS: 1-2

INGREDIENTS

SALAD
1 tin tuna shredded or chunks, drained
1 soft-boiled egg, finely chopped
1/2 cup halved cherry tomatoes
1/2 avocado, diced or sliced
1/2 red onion finely sliced or diced
1/2 cup grated carrot or zucchini or similar
1/2 cup cooked pasta or chickpeas (optional)

DRESSING
1 tablespoon mayo or plain yogurt
1 teaspoon mustard
pinch lemon zest
pinch black pepper
2 tablespoons water

TO SERVE
1/2 head romaine, iceberg or cos lettuce

METHOD

Let's face it: tinned tuna is a necessary evil.
Yes, I prefer fresh but sometimes it just isn't available and you need to reach for the tin.
It's always handy to know how to pimp up a tin of tuna.

Place the drained tuna and all the ingredients into a large bowl and mix to combine.
Stir the dressing through and then season to taste.
You can then serve this over the lettuce leaves, or have it just on it's own.
For a hit of glamour, use a stacking ring to give it height and that 'Wow!' factor.
Delicious and packed with goodness.

Sauces & Dressings

Add some delicious flavour.

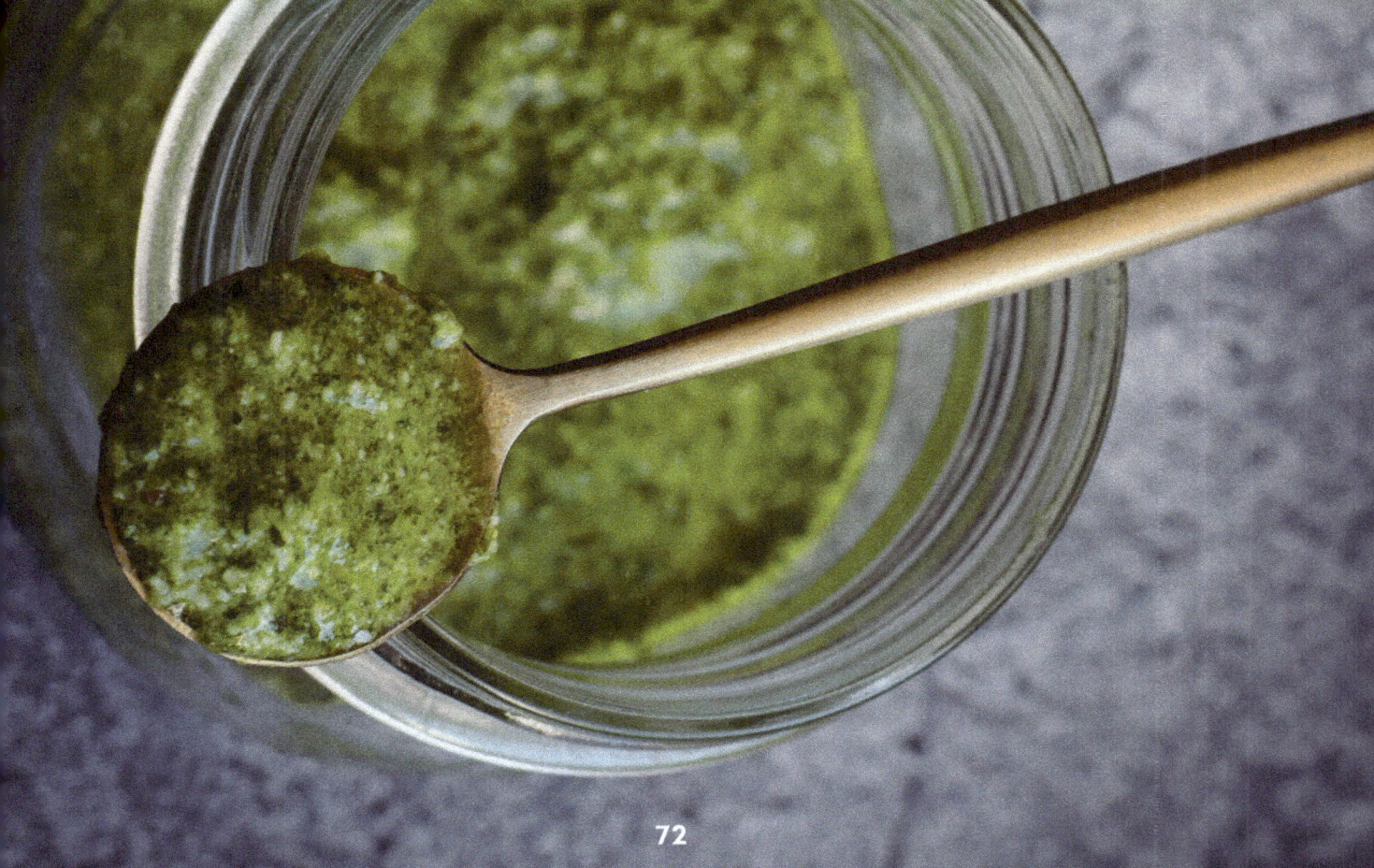

Carrot Ginger Dressing

SERVINGS: 2-4

INGREDIENTS

1 carrot, peeled and roughly cut
1 tablespoon ginger, peeled and cut roughly
1 tablespoon cider or your favourite vinegar
3 tablespoons oil
Drop sesame oil

METHOD

Blend in your smoothie maker until this forms a bright orange velvety dressing. You really do need a blender for this, please don't make this without one, it just won't be the same.
Perfect on salads, over leftover vegetables or any dish at all.

Asian Style Dressing

SERVINGS: 2-4

INGREDIENTS

1/4 cup fish sauce
4 tablespoons rice vinegar
2 tablespoons white sugar
1/2 cup warm water
2 garlic cloves, crushed
3 red Birdseye chilli
3 tablespoons lime juice

METHOD

To make your dressing, simply place ingredients together in a jar or a clean bottle, put a closely fitting lid on and shake or stir to combine.
With this dressing, you are wanting sweet, sour and hot.
Season to taste. It can be stored for a month in the fridge.
Perfect over-cooked chicken, seafood or veggies...will add some spice and happiness to many dishes.
I especially love this dressing over rare roast beef or even roasted pumpkin with lots of freshly chopped coriander/cilantro.

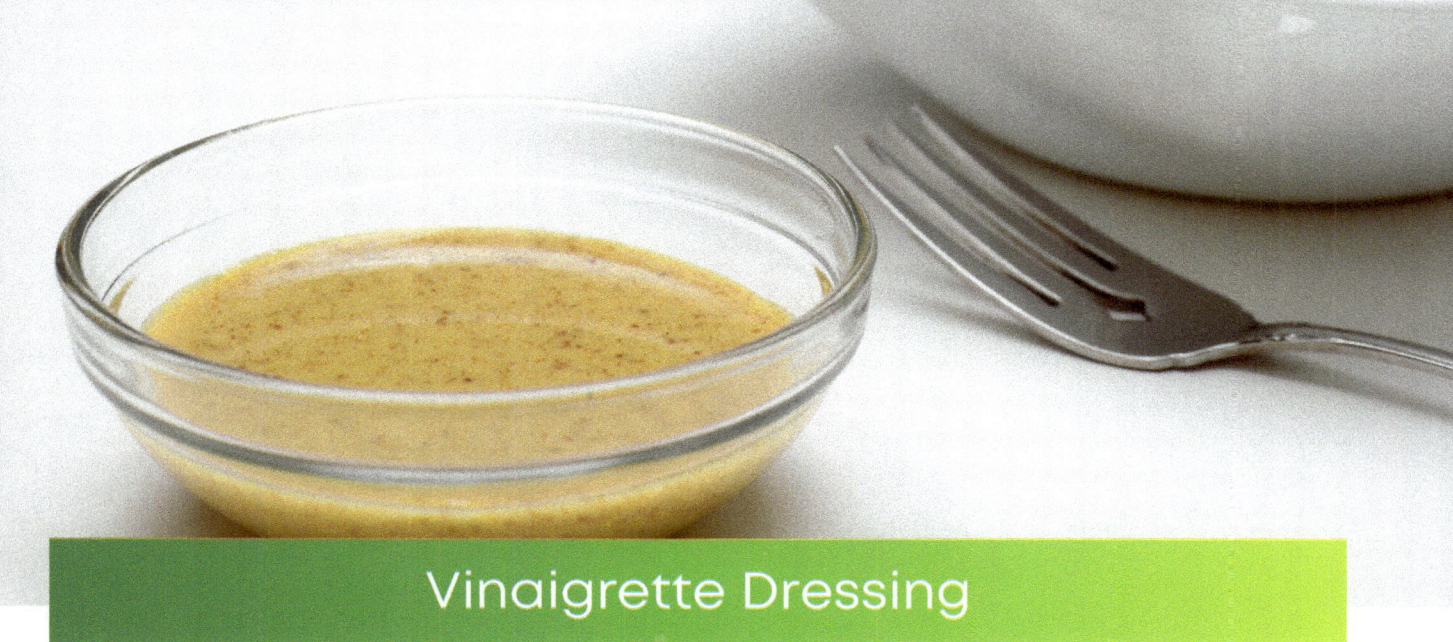

Vinaigrette Dressing

SERVINGS: 2-4

INGREDIENTS

50 ml good vinegar or lemon juice
150 ml Extra Virgin Olive oil or your choice of vegetable oil
1 tablespoon of your choice of mustard
1 tablespoon finely chopped or minced shallots or onion
1 tablespoon finely parsley, basil, thyme or your favourite

METHOD

The easiest way to make the most traditional salad dressing, the vinaigrette, is to remember your ratios. This will mean you can rehash this recipe again and again for many years to come, and you'll always be confident making it.

The standard ratio is one part vinegar/lemon juice to three parts oil. Then we add our seasoning, depending on what you are dressing. Generally, this is seasoned by using mustard, herbs and spices.

Try to use the best vinegar you have, white balsamic or those fancy berry or wine vinegars are the best. For the oil, you can use your favourite, either an olive oil or a vegetable oil of your choosing. As always, use fresh oils that are in date, please don't ever use rancid or stale oil!
To make your vinaigrette, simply place ingredients together in a jar or a clean bottle, put a closely fitting lid on and shake or stir to combine.

Season to taste. It can be stored for a month in the fridge.

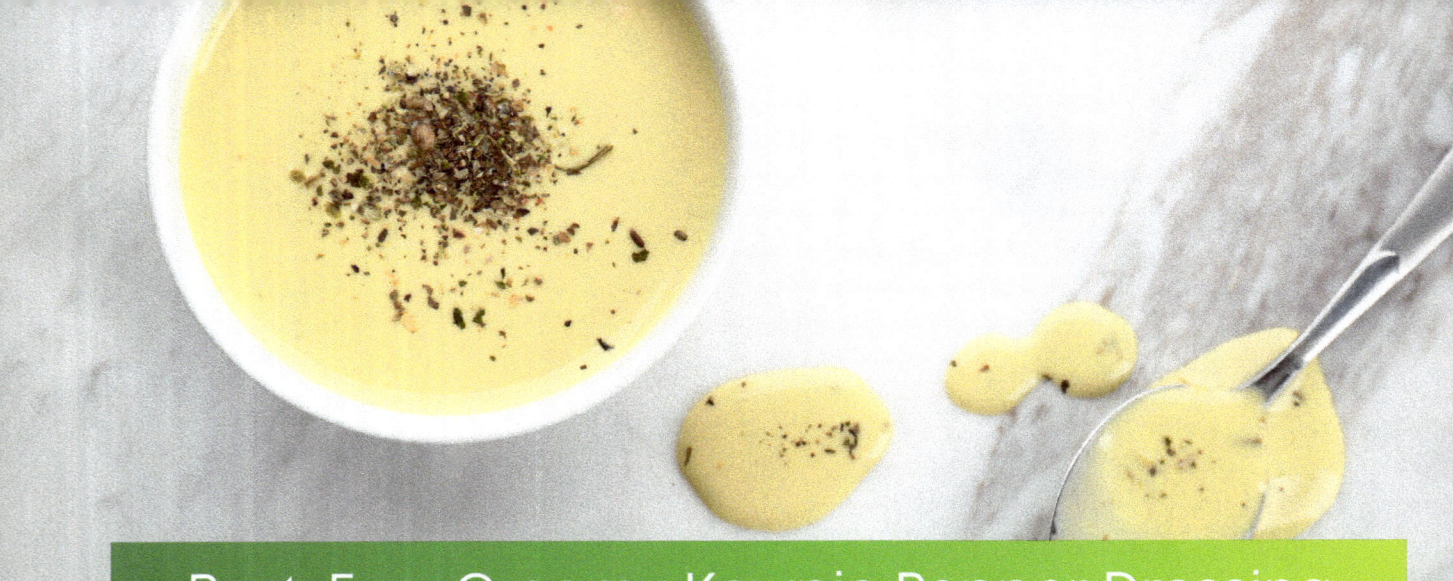

Best-Ever Creamy Kewpie Pepper Dressing

SERVINGS: 2-4

INGREDIENTS

4 tablespoons Kewpie or Whole Egg Mayo
1/2 teaspoon cracked or freshly ground black pepper
80ml cold water

METHOD

This dressing is extremely versatile and very quick and easy to make.

Place all of your ingredients into the jar you plan to serve this from. If you are making this for later, simply store in an airtight container for up to 2 weeks in the fridge. You can make it as you need it, or double or triple this recipe if you end up using it as much as I do.
So sexy and quick and cheap and easy! I use this dressing over salads, chicken breast, corn, or anything that needs a bit of creamy pepper dressing.

VARIATIONS

You can change the flavour combinations of this dressing as many times as you like.
Try adding the zest and juice of a lemon for fish and seafood dishes.
Or add half a teaspoon of fresh curry powder or Ras el Hanout spices to use as a dreamy spiced dressing.
Add toasted sesame seeds and a few drops of sesame seed oil to create a fantastic zing to hundreds of dishes.
I also add orange zest and juice. Make this your own way.

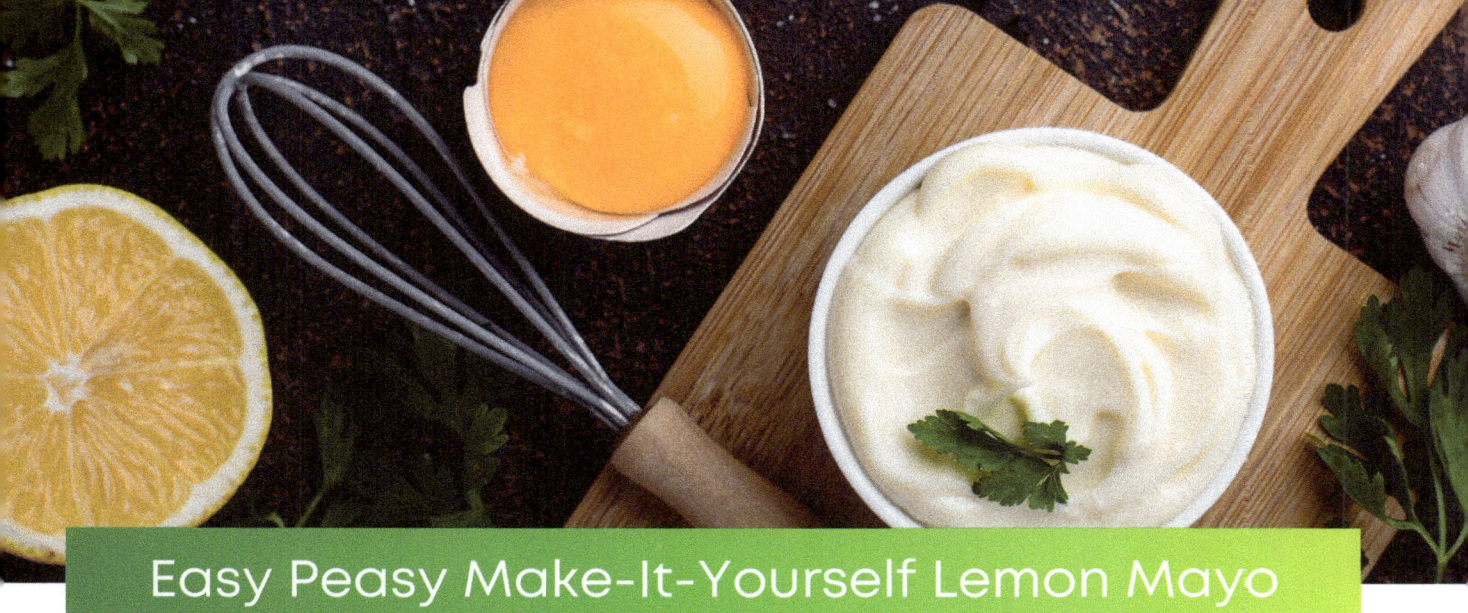

Easy Peasy Make-It-Yourself Lemon Mayo

SERVINGS: 8-10

INGREDIENTS

(MAKES JUST OVER 350ML)
1 egg yolk, at room temperature
Big pinch salt
5ml Dijon or other mustard
Pinch black coarsely ground pepper
Zest of one lemon
15ml lemon juice
300ml sunflower/canola/rice bran oil

METHOD

Place the egg yolk into a blender, or if you're doing this by hand, into a large wide-mouthed bowl.

Add the big pinch of salt, black pepper, lemon juice zest and mustard and blend or whisk together.

Now you can pop the blender on a low setting and pour the 300 ml oil in a thin, steady stream until the mixture starts to thicken. If you are beating by hand, put a wet cloth under the bowl so it doesn't move around, and then whisk quickly, pouring the oil in a thin stream and whisking to incorporate it into the egg mix. It will go lovely and thick and creamy.

Adjust seasoning and serve, or store in the fridge for up to one week.

You can swap the lemon juice for white balsamic vinegar if you prefer!

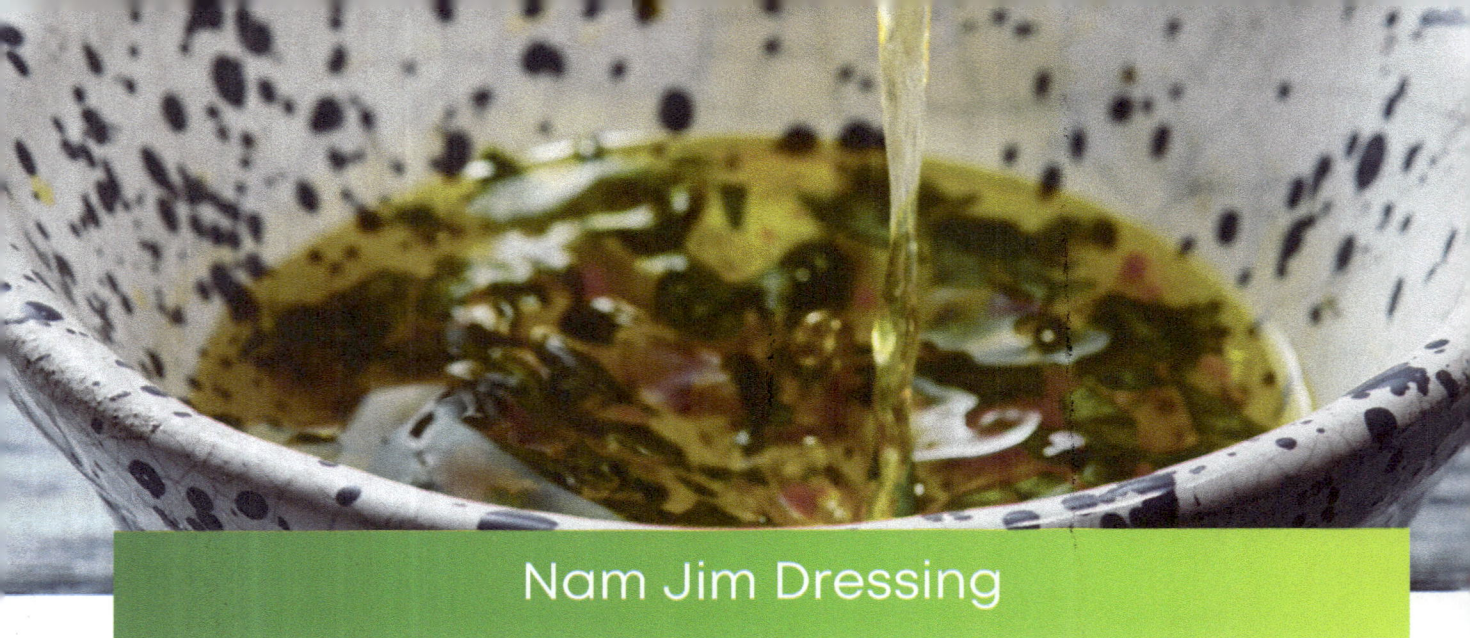

Nam Jim Dressing

SERVINGS: 4-6

INGREDIENTS

2 tablespoons chopped red shallot or onion
1 tablespoon finely chopped spring onion
1 tablespoon finely chopped coriander/cilantro
1 tablespoon crushed ginger
1 garlic clove, crushed
2 tablespoons tamarind paste
1 tablespoon brown sugar, sweetener or maple syrup
2 tablespoons fish sauce
1 tablespoon warm water
1/2 teaspoon chilli powder (more or less according to taste)
1 teaspoon roasted rice
1 teaspoon roasted sesame seeds ground

METHOD

To roast the rice and sesame seeds, place them into a dry frying pan and place over the heat.
Shake until the rice and the sesame seeds are brown and fragrant.
When they are cool, bash down in your pestle and mortar, or place in the blender.

Add the remaining ingredients and either blend or stir together.
You can use this as a salad dressing, marinade or stir-fry sauce.

So delicious! Make it as hot as you like with the chilli.

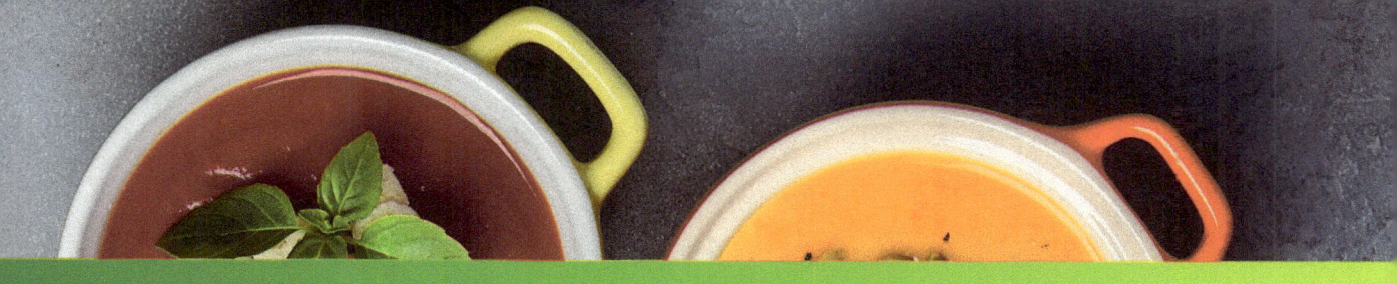

Soups

These healthy soup recipes are delicious and packed with nutrients. They can be a satisfying meal on their own or served alongside a salad or whole-grain bread for a complete and nourishing meal.

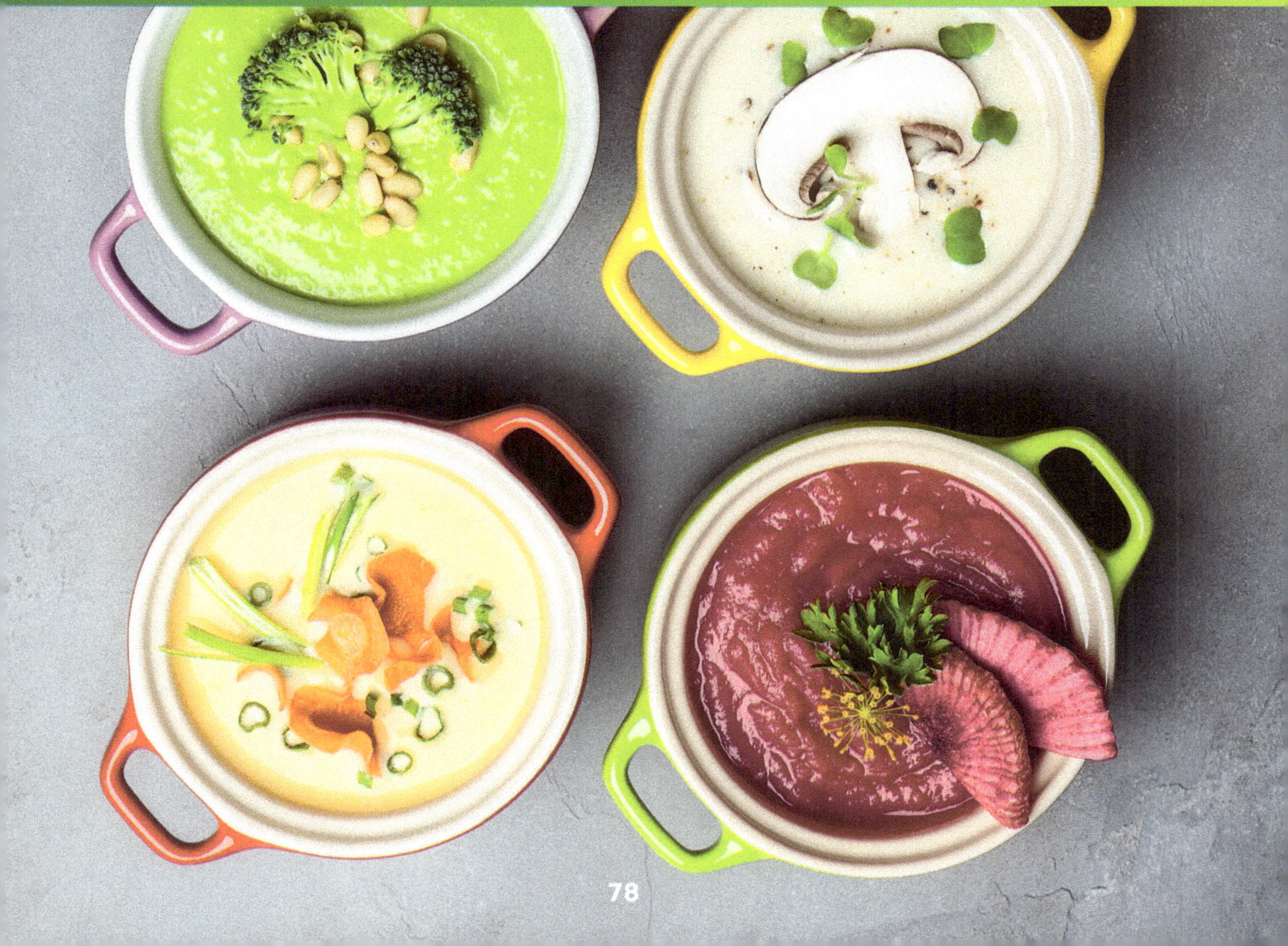

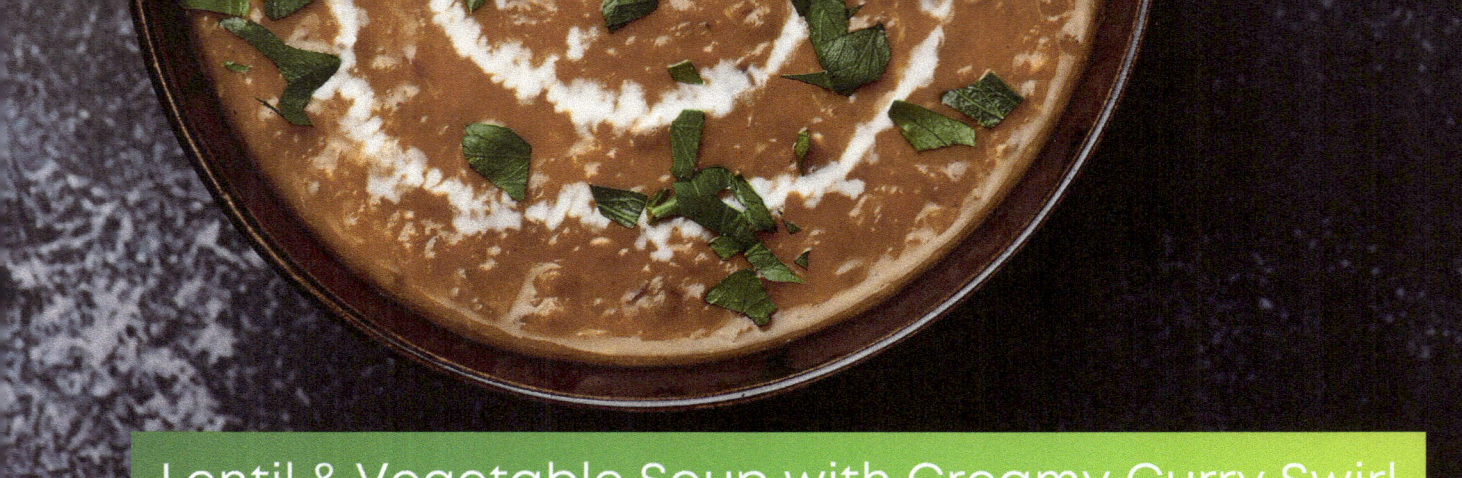

Lentil & Vegetable Soup with Creamy Curry Swirl

SERVINGS: 4-6

INGREDIENTS

SOUP

- 2 tablespoons olive oil
- 1 cup dried lentils, or use a tin if you're in a hurry
- 1 large onion, diced
- 2 carrots, diced
- 2 celery stalks, diced
- 1 zucchini or other veggies your choice, diced
- 1 can diced tomatoes
- 1 litre vegetable stock
- 2 cloves garlic, minced
- 1 teaspoon fresh or dried thyme
- 1 teaspoon fresh or dried oregano
- Salt and pepper to taste

CREAMY CURRY SWIRL

- 50 ml dairy or coconut cream
- 1/2 teaspoon Ras el Hanout or curry powder or just use cumin and coriander/cilantro

METHOD

Heat olive oil in a large pot over medium heat. Add onions, carrots, celery, and garlic. Sauté until softened.

Add lentils, zucchini, diced tomatoes, thyme, oregano, salt, and pepper. Stir to combine.

Pour in vegetable broth and bring the soup to a boil. Reduce heat, cover, and let it simmer for about 20-25 minutes until the lentils are tender.

When cooked, adjust the seasoning and then either serve rustic with the chunks OR you can use your stick blender with the metal head to get this into a glorious thick velvety soup.

Plate up and then just before serving, garnish with a swirl of the creamy curry swirl.

You can also top with chopped chilli and coriander.

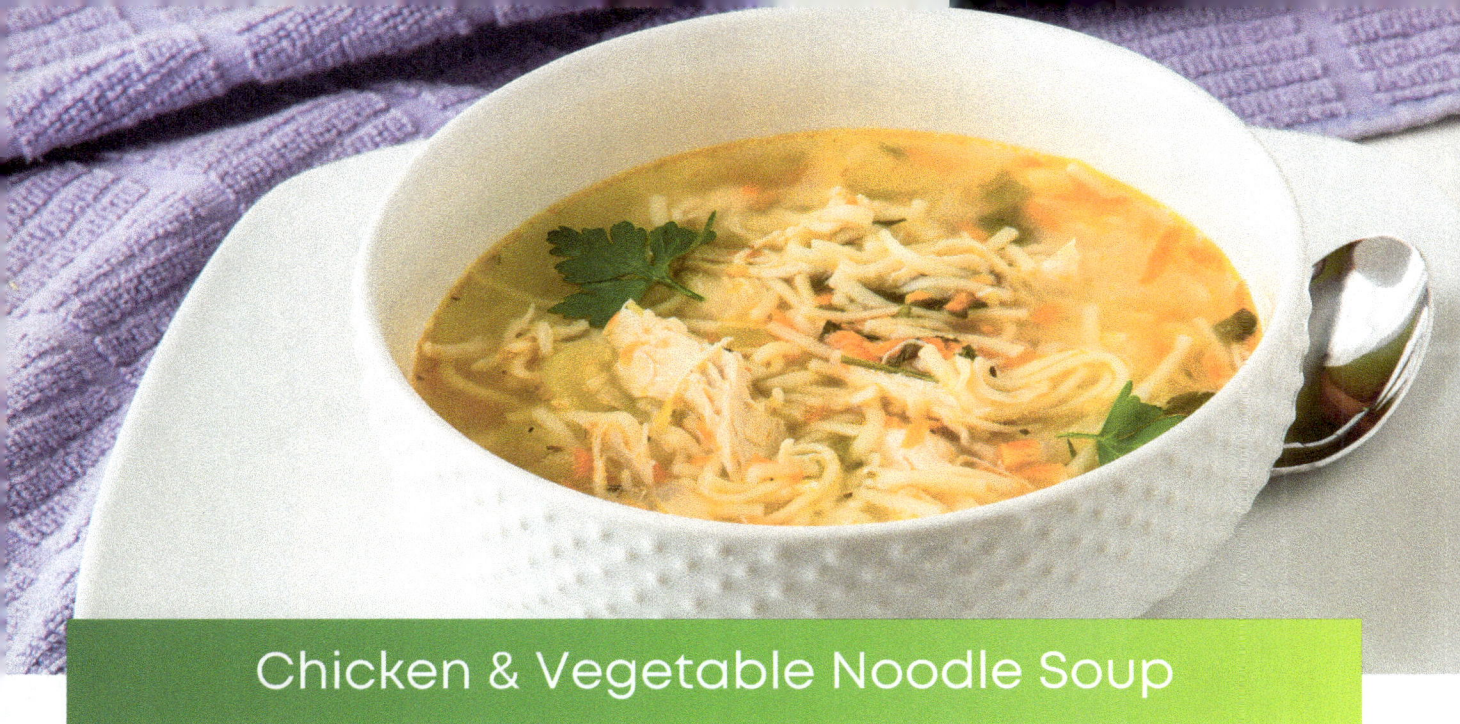

Chicken & Vegetable Noodle Soup

SERVINGS: 4-6

INGREDIENTS

1-litre vegetable or chicken stock
2 boneless skinless chicken breasts or you can use 1 small whole chicken
1 onion, finely chopped
1 cup chopped zucchini
1 cup sliced white mushrooms
1 cup sliced carrots
2 cloves garlic, minced
2 tablespoons soy sauce
1 tablespoon grated ginger
1 cup cooked rice noodles or whole wheat noodles (store-bought is perfect)
Fresh coriander/cilantro, chopped chilli and green onions for garnish

METHOD

In a large pot, bring the stock to a simmer.
Add shredded chicken, onions, mushrooms, zucchini, carrots, garlic, soy sauce, and ginger.
Stir to combine.
Cook the soup on low heat for about 15-20 minutes until the vegetables are tender.
Meanwhile, cook the rice or whole wheat noodles according to the package instructions.
Once the vegetables are tender, add the cooked noodles to the soup and stir. Adjust the seasoning.
Garnish with fresh coriander/cilantro, chilli and green onions before serving.

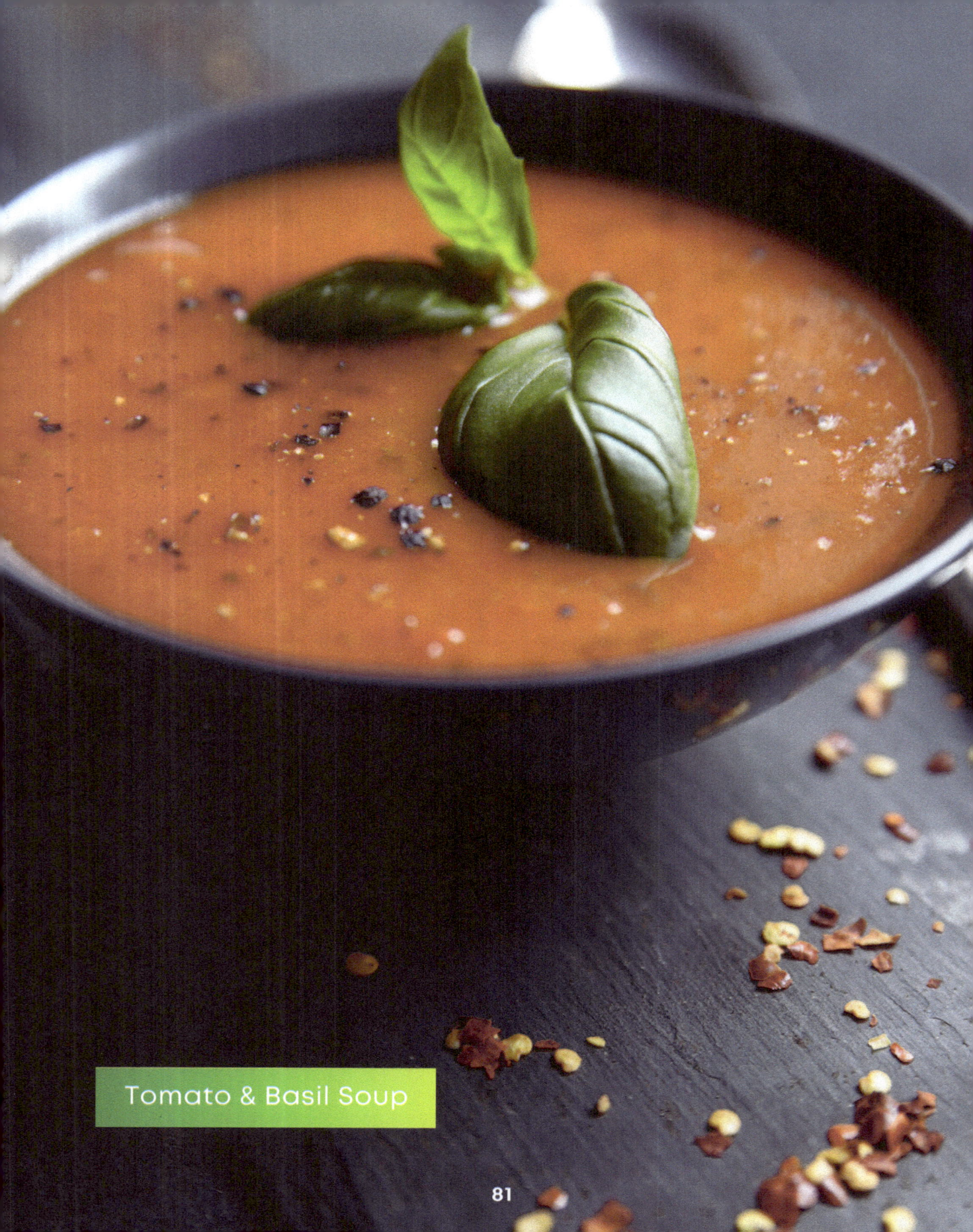
Tomato & Basil Soup

Tomato & Basil Soup

SERVINGS: 4-6

INGREDIENTS

CAN BE SERVED HOT OR COLD

1 tablespoon olive oil
1 large onion, diced
2 cloves garlic, minced
2 tins canned tomatoes (440g / 15 oz each)
1 cup vegetable stock, well seasoned
1/4 cup fresh basil leaves, chopped
Salt and pepper to taste

METHOD

In a large pot, heat olive oil over medium heat. Add onions and garlic, and sauté until translucent. Add canned tomatoes and vegetable stock and then bring to a boil.

Reduce heat and let it simmer for about 10 minutes.

Use a stick blender with a metal head or transfer the soup to a blender, (wait until the soup is cold if the blender is sealed like a bullet blender) then pulse or blend to puree until smooth.
Season to taste, use lots of freshly ground black pepper and salt.

Serve hot or cold, garnished a fresh drizzle of extra virgin olive oil and with a few fresh basil leaves

"Cooking is all about people. Food is maybe the only universal thing that really has the power to bring everyone together. No matter what culture, everywhere around the world, people get together to eat."
— Guy Fieri

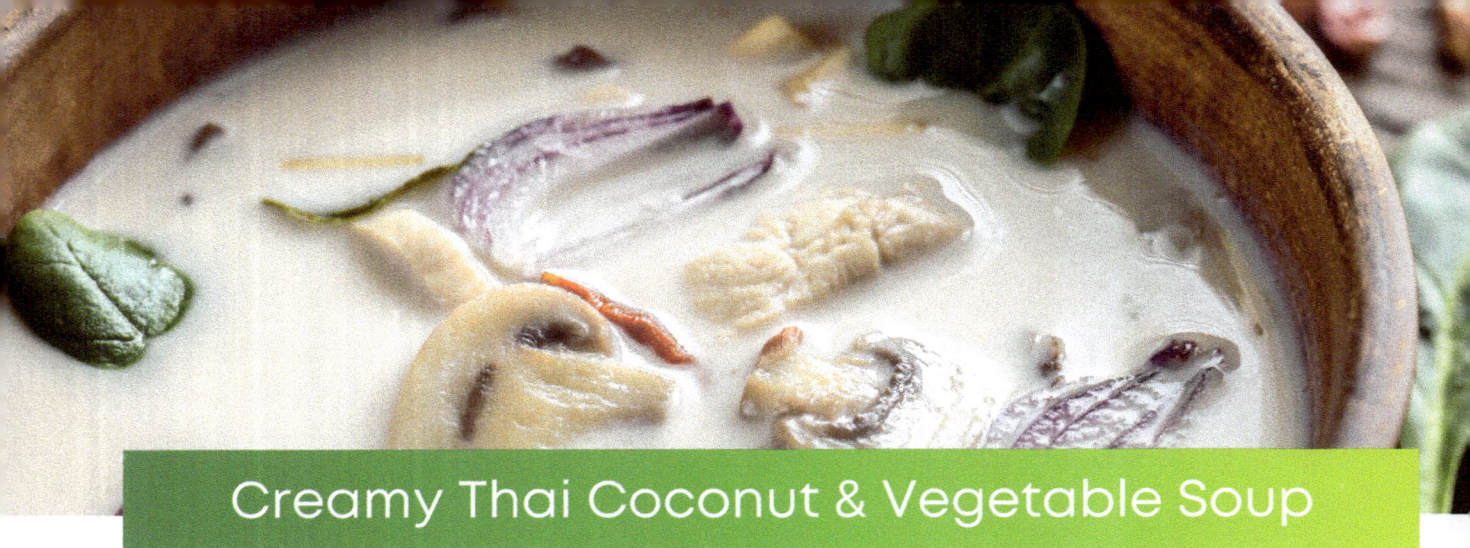

Creamy Thai Coconut & Vegetable Soup

SERVINGS: 4-6

INGREDIENTS

1 tablespoon coconut oil
1 onion, diced
2 cloves garlic, minced
1 tablespoon grated ginger
1 red bell pepper, thinly sliced
1 cup sliced mushrooms
1 small can of coconut milk or cream
1-litre vegetable or chicken stock
2 tablespoons soy sauce
1 tablespoon Thai red curry paste (adjust to taste)
Juice of 1 lime
Fresh coriander/cilantro and sliced green onions for garnish

METHOD

In a large pot, heat coconut oil over medium heat.
Add onions, garlic, and grated ginger. Sauté until aromatic.

Add sliced red bell pepper and mushrooms. Cook for a few minutes until they start to soften.
Pour in coconut milk, vegetable broth, soy sauce, and Thai red curry paste.
Stir well to dissolve the curry paste.

Bring the soup to a simmer and cook for about 10-15 minutes, allowing the flavours to meld together.
Just before serving, add lime juice and stir.
Garnish with fresh coriander/cilantro and sliced green onions.

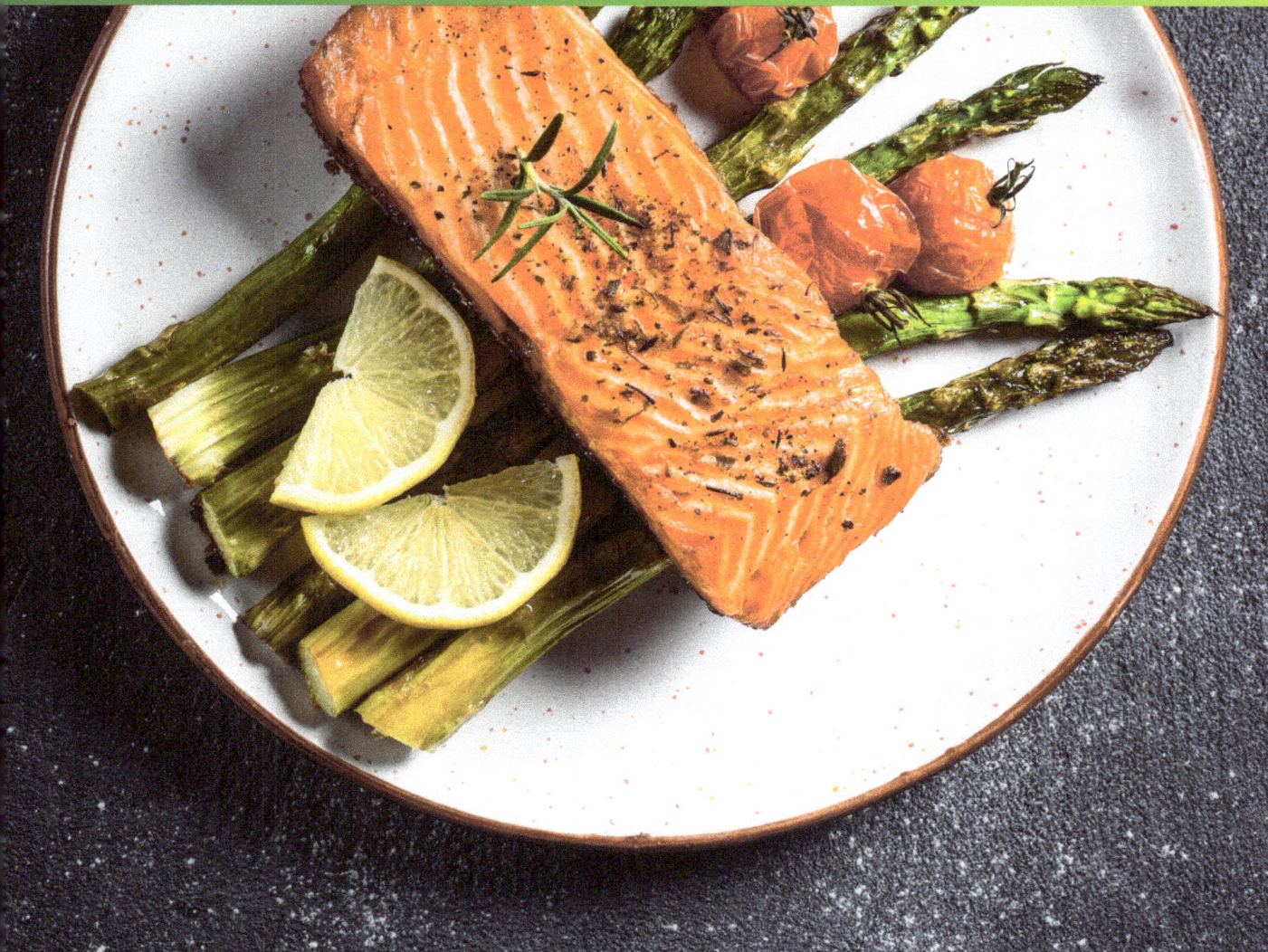

Mains

For family dinners or dinner parties.

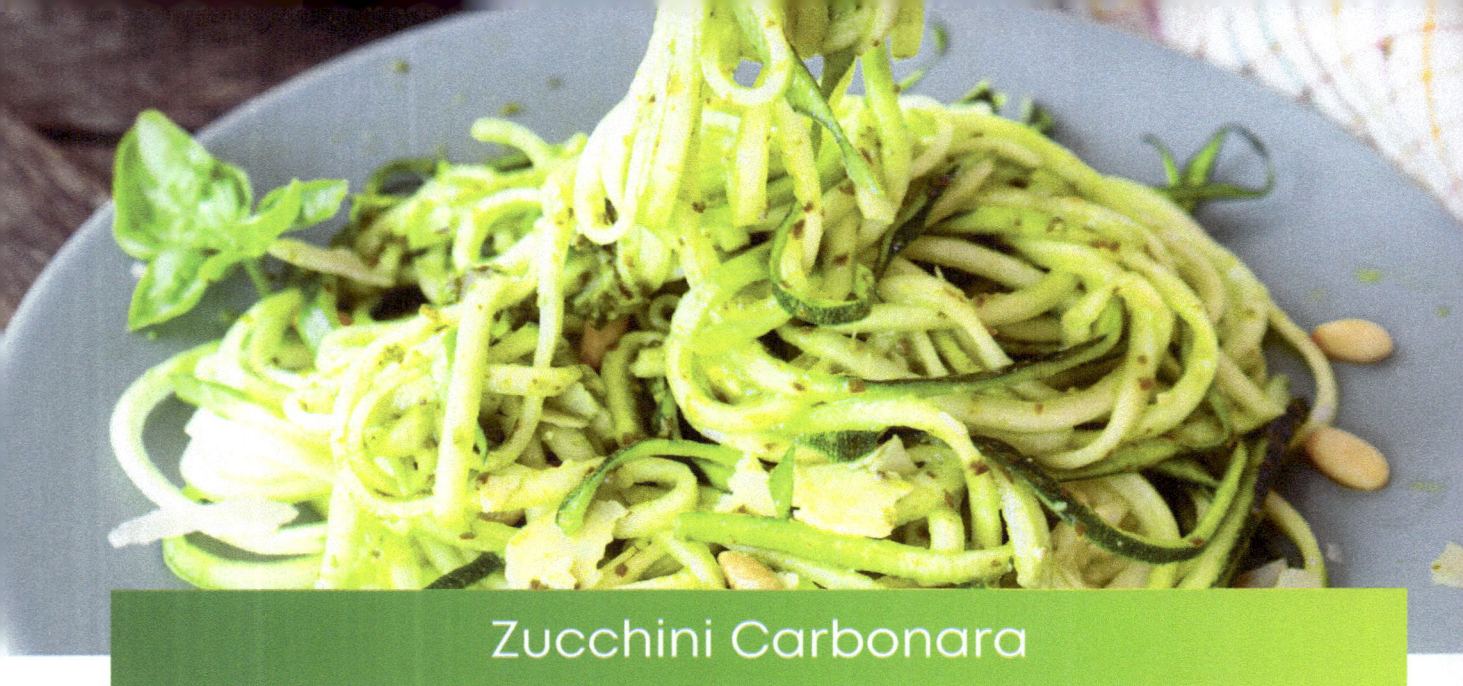

Zucchini Carbonara

SERVINGS: 1-2

INGREDIENTS

1 clove garlic, crushed
2-3 rashers bacon, streaky or other
1 large zucchini cut into ribbons with a veggie peeler, or use a veggie spiralizer.
2 eggs, beaten with 50 ml water
1 tablespoon chopped parsley, chives, basil or sage - you choose!
1 tablespoon grated or shaved Parmesan or Pecorino

METHOD

Heat and grease the frying pan well, use a canola or rice bran or veggie oil.

Place the diced bacon in the pan and let the bacon go crisp and brown and flavoursome. You want to render all the fat off, that is where the flavour is after all.

Add the raw zucchini ribbons into the pan and stir fry until just tender and heated through. No need to overcook.

Remove from the heat and place on a heat-proof surface. Get two chopsticks or a fork, and stir the egg and water through, stirring as you go. The residual heat will slowly thicken the egg as you stir.

Once nice and thick you can season with the cheese and then serve with cracked pepper.

Zucchini Bolognaise

SERVINGS: 6-8

INGREDIENTS

Cooking spray or little vegetable oil to grease the pan

1kg premium beef mince

1 large onion finely sliced

3-6 cloves garlic

3 tablespoons fresh oregano/thyme/marjoram *or use 1 teaspoon dried Italian herb mix*

1 carrot, finely diced or grated

1 celery stalk, finely grated

1 pinch nutmeg (very important!)

80ml milk (optional)

2-3 teaspoons beef stock powder or 2 stock cubes

1 tin chopped tomatoes

1 jar passata (500-700ml)

4 large zucchini, spiralized into noodles

(you can use your peeler and make ribbons, or use a spiralizer tool)

METHOD

Heat and grease a large pan until it is just about smoking hot.

Now add the mince that you have broken up in the packaging or a bowl so it is loose and fluffy already. Put the mince into the pan. IT SHOULD SIZZLE nice and loud and sexy.

DO NOT STIR, I know you are worried about this burning and you are also worried about lumps, but let the mince brown and seal on the first side you put down FIRST and let the pan heat up again and THEN you can stir ever so slightly just to get some more mince onto the base of the pan. My favourite mince 'fluffer' is one of those cheap plastic-coated whisks you get at the supermarket that only have about 4 loops. If you don't have one of those use a strong plastic spoon or egg flip to break down the mince.

Once the mince is brown and fragrant and sexy ALL BY ITSELF, then and only then, do you add the finely chopped onion and garlic. There should be a good amount of fat rendered out of the mince during your amazing sizzling at a nice high heat.

You can stir as much as you like now by the way. That mince is SEALED off!

Now add the herbs, milk, nutmeg, stock powder, grated/diced carrot and seasoning and stir through. Amazing colour isn't it?

Finally, add the chopped tomatoes, vegetables and passata and you're practically done. Turn down the heat and let that all cook through and then check the seasoning and it's ready to serve.

This way of cooking will not only save you time, BUT it will add valuable flavour and vibrant personality to your otherwise boring mince.

Serve with stir-fried zucchini ribbons, shaved parmesan and lots of freshly chopped parsley.

Mel's Note: I love to get creative with my mince and change the spices, thus changing the flavour.

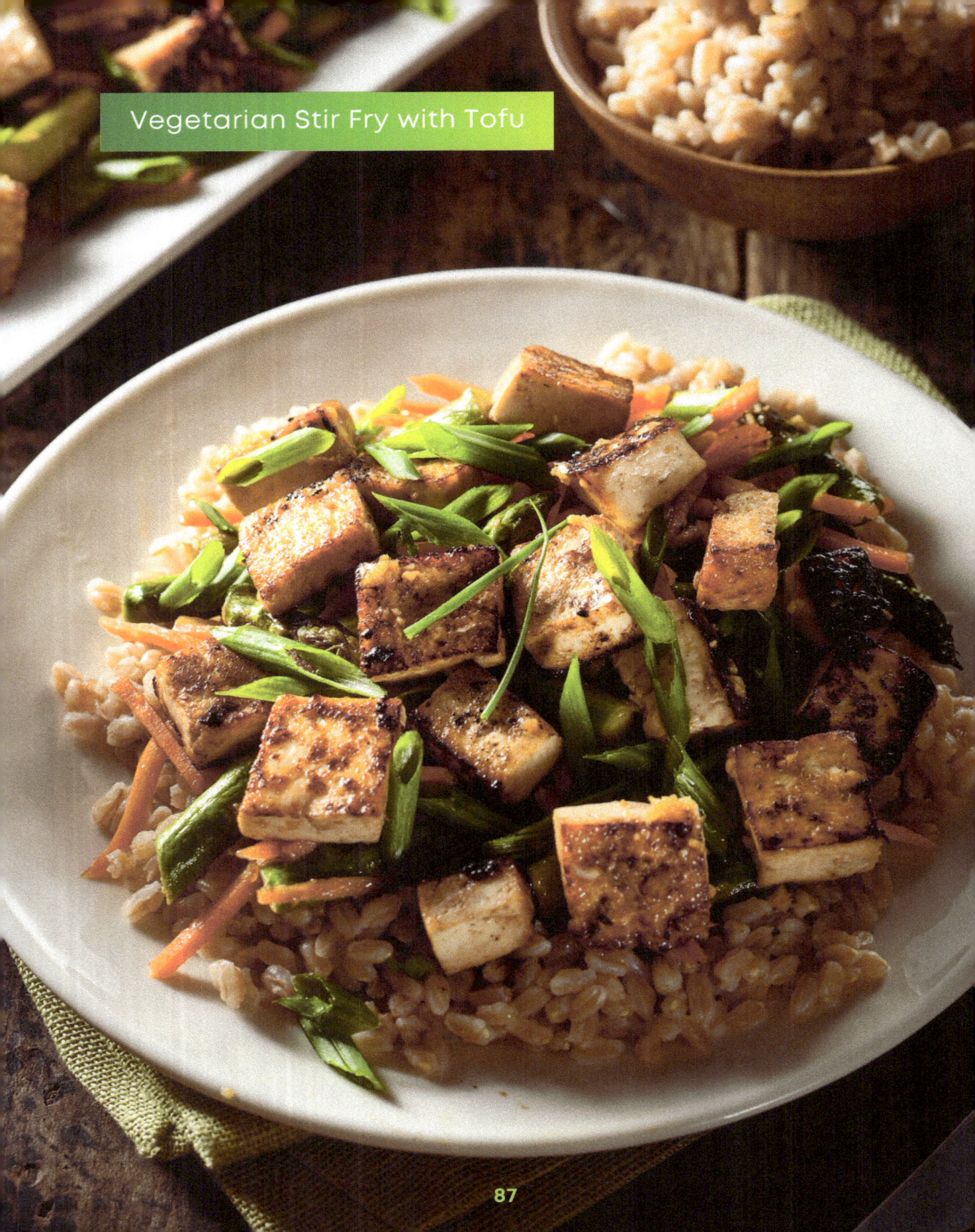

Vegetarian Stir Fry with Tofu

Vegetarian Stir Fry with Tofu

SERVINGS: 2-4

INGREDIENTS

1 block firm tofu, drained and cubed
2 tablespoons soy sauce
2 tablespoons hoisin sauce
1 tablespoon sesame oil (please make sure it's fresh)
2 tablespoons vegetable oil
1 onion, thinly sliced
1 red capsicum/pepper, thinly sliced
1 yellow capsicum/pepper, thinly sliced
1 cup broccoli florets
1 cup snow peas
2 cloves garlic, minced
1-inch piece of fresh ginger, grated
2 green onions, sliced
Sesame seeds for garnish (optional)
Cooked brown rice or quinoa for serving

METHOD

In a bowl, marinate the cubed tofu with soy sauce and hoisin sauce for about 10-15 minutes.

In a wok or large non-stick frying pan, heat the sesame oil and vegetable oil over medium-high heat.
Add the marinated tofu to the wok and stir fry until lightly browned.
Remove from the wok and set aside.
In the same wok, stir fry the sliced onion and capsicum/peppers for a few minutes until slightly softened.
Add the broccoli, snap peas, garlic, and ginger to the wok.
Stir fry for another 3-4 minutes until the vegetables are tender-crisp.

Return the tofu to the wok and toss everything together.
Sprinkle with sliced green onions and sesame seeds before serving over brown rice or quinoa.

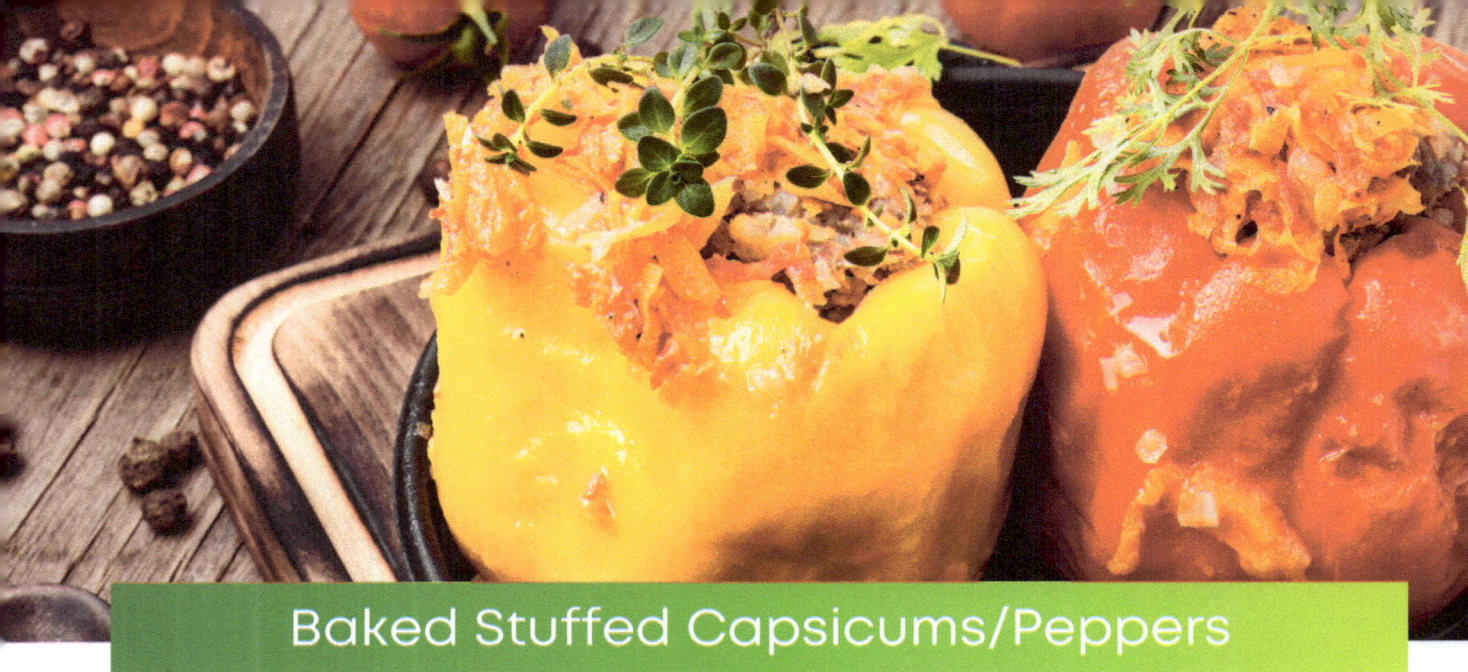

Baked Stuffed Capsicums/Peppers

SERVINGS: 4

INGREDIENTS

4 large capsicums/ peppers (any color)
1 cup cooked, shredded chicken, cooked mince or any other protein
1 cup cooked quinoa or brown rice
1 can black beans, drained and rinsed
1 cup diced tomatoes
1 cup corn kernels, fresh or frozen
1 teaspoon chili powder
1/2 teaspoon cumin
Salt and pepper to taste (always season well)
1/2 cup shredded cheddar cheese (optional)

METHOD

Preheat the oven to 200C, nice and hot.
Cut the tops off the bell peppers and remove the seeds and membranes.
In a bowl, mix together the cooked quinoa, cooked protein, black beans, diced tomatoes, corn, chili powder, cumin, salt, and pepper.
Stuff each bell pepper with the quinoa mixture and place them in a baking dish.
If using cheese, sprinkle the shredded cheddar on top of each stuffed pepper.
Cover the baking dish with foil and bake for about 30-35 minutes until the peppers are tender.
Remove the foil and bake for an additional 5 minutes to melt the cheese (if using).
I love these for dinner parties or just a week night meal.
You can use any filling you like.

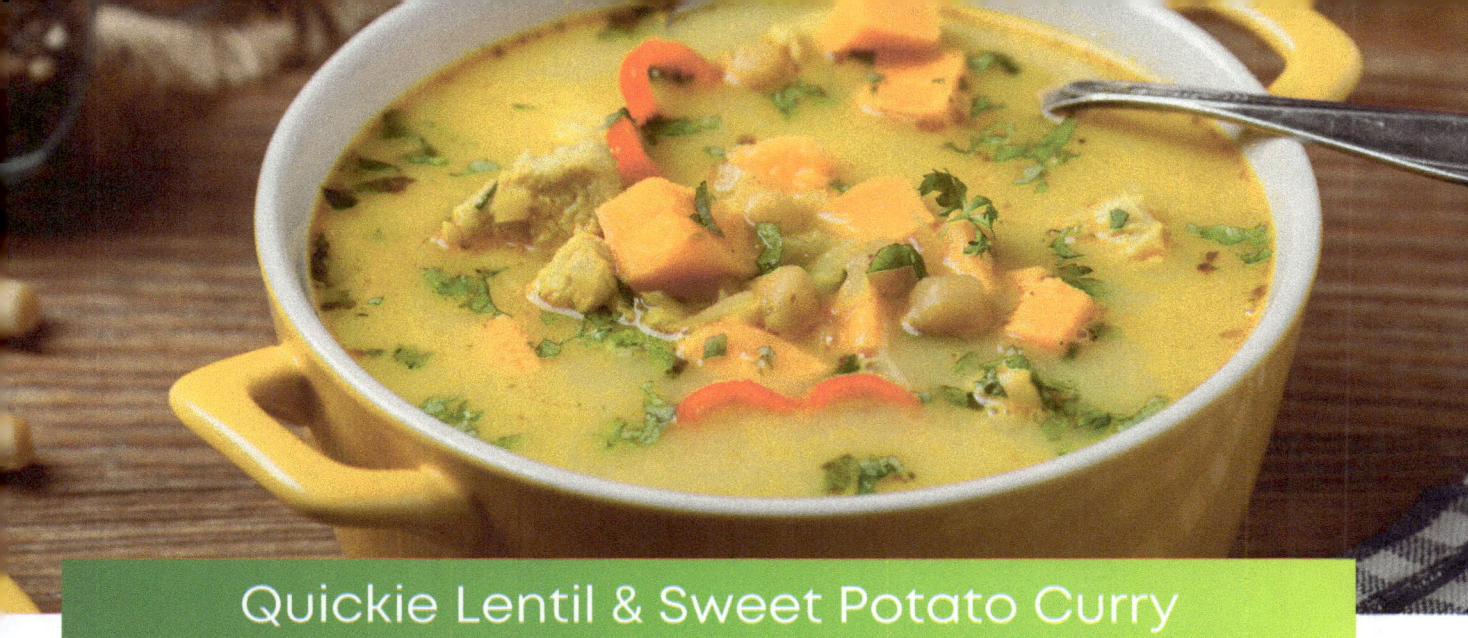

Quickie Lentil & Sweet Potato Curry

SERVINGS: 2

INGREDIENTS

1 tin lentils, drained
1 large sweet potato, peeled and diced and cooked in microwave or air fryer until tender.
1 onion, finely diced
2 cloves garlic, minced
1 tablespoon grated ginger
1 can of coconut milk
1 can diced tomatoes
2 tablespoons curry powder
1 teaspoon ground cumin
1/2 teaspoon turmeric
Salt and pepper to taste
Fresh coriander/cilantro for garnish
Cooked brown rice or quinoa for serving

METHOD

In a large pot, sauté the diced onion, garlic, and grated ginger until fragrant and softened.
Add the lentils, diced sweet potato, coconut milk, diced tomatoes, curry powder, cumin, turmeric, salt, and pepper to the pot. Stir to combine.
Bring the mixture to a boil, then reduce the heat, cover, and let it simmer for about 15-20 minutes or until the lentils are tender. Add the sweet potatoes and warm through.
Adjust seasoning if necessary and serve the lentil and sweet potato curry over cooked brown rice or quinoa.
Garnish with fresh coriander/cilantro.

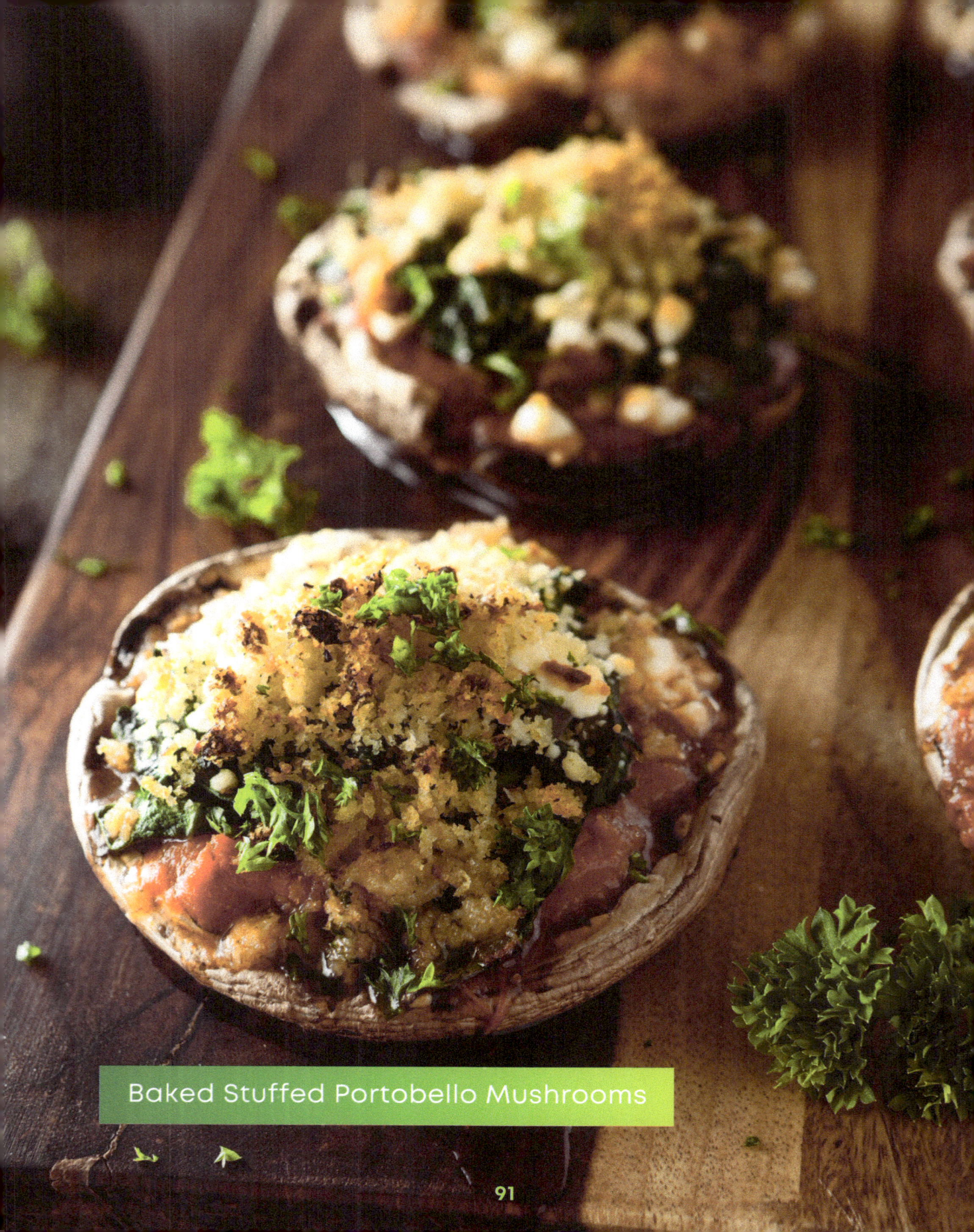
Baked Stuffed Portobello Mushrooms

Baked Stuffed Portobello Mushrooms

SERVINGS: 4

INGREDIENTS

4 large portobello mushrooms, stems removed and gills scraped out
1 cup cooked quinoa or couscous
1 cup chopped spinach
1/2 cup crumbled feta cheese
1/4 cup chopped sun-dried tomatoes
2 cloves garlic, minced
2 tablespoons olive oil
Salt and pepper to taste
Fresh parsley for garnish

METHOD

Preheat the oven to 200C and then line a baking sheet with baking paper.
In a bowl, mix together the cooked quinoa or couscous, chopped spinach, crumbled feta cheese, sun-dried tomatoes, minced garlic, olive oil, salt, and pepper.
Stuff each portobello mushroom cap with the quinoa mixture and place them on the prepared baking sheet.
Bake for about 15-20 minutes until the mushrooms are tender and the filling is heated through.
Garnish with fresh parsley before serving.

"Cooking and baking is both physical and mental therapy."
— Mary Berry

Truffled Mushroom 'Pizza' with Cauli & Sweet Potato Topping

SERVINGS: 4-6

INGREDIENTS

4-6 large brown mushrooms, wrapped in greased foil to protect them in the oven
1 cup cauliflower mash
(simply simmer cauli in milk and/or stock until tender, season and then mash)
1 cup roasted sweet potato slices
2 tablespoons truffle/lemon/orange oil (from deli or supermarket)
Salt and pepper to season
Parmesan cheese finely grated on zester to make Parmesan snow

METHOD

Top the mushroom with the roasted sweet potato and then the cauli, drizzle with the oil and then garnish with the cheese, bake for about 10-12 minutes in a hot oven (200C) until done…delicious!

"Cooking is about passion, so it may look slightly temperamental in a way that it's too assertive to the naked eye."
— Gordon Ramsay

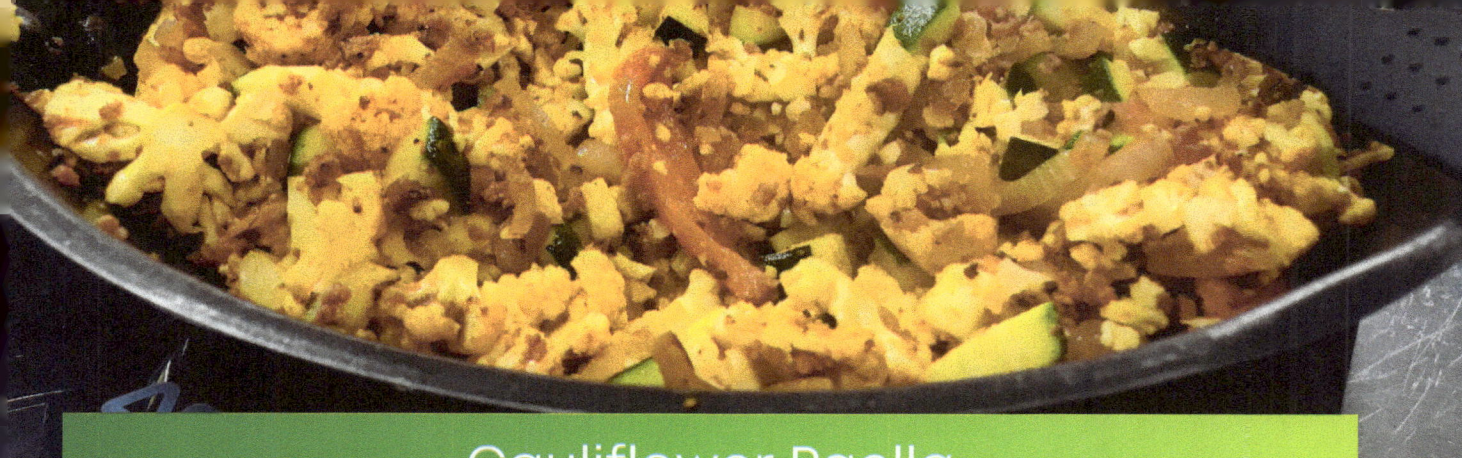

Cauliflower Paella

SERVINGS: 4

INGREDIENTS

10ml oil or cooking spray
450-600g chicken pieces of your choice
cut into pieces no larger than your palm (optional, you can keep this vegetarian)
80g chorizo sausage or bacon, finely diced or minced *(optional)*
1 onion, minced or finely chopped
1 head cauliflower, food processed (cauliflower rice)
1 tablespoon smoked or sweet Paprika
1 teaspoon ground turmeric
1 teaspoon garlic paste
1 teaspoon chicken stock powder
Juice and zest of one lemon
1 cup peas, snow peas or beans
80g fire-roasted capsicum (from your deli)
Pinch of dried or 1 teaspoon of fresh sage or thyme

METHOD

Spray a large nonstick frying pan with cooking spray or oil and allow the pan to get swearword hot. Once hot add the chorizo gravel/mince and allow to brown nicely. Don't stir just for fun, only stir if it needs to be stirred! We want the sausage to render its fat and if you cool it down too much it will stew.
Now add the onions, garlic, and herbs and cook through. You can reduce the heat at this stage.
Coat the chicken in the spices and the stock powder to give it a Spanish spray tan. Make some space in the pan, turn the heat up, and add the chicken to the hot pan. Don't stir until the first layer of chicken is brown, then stir and turn the pieces to brown.
Once browned, add the capsicum, peas, cauliflower rice and lemon zest, and stir fry until tender.
Season to taste and then add the lemon juice!
Ready to serve! So quick and easy!

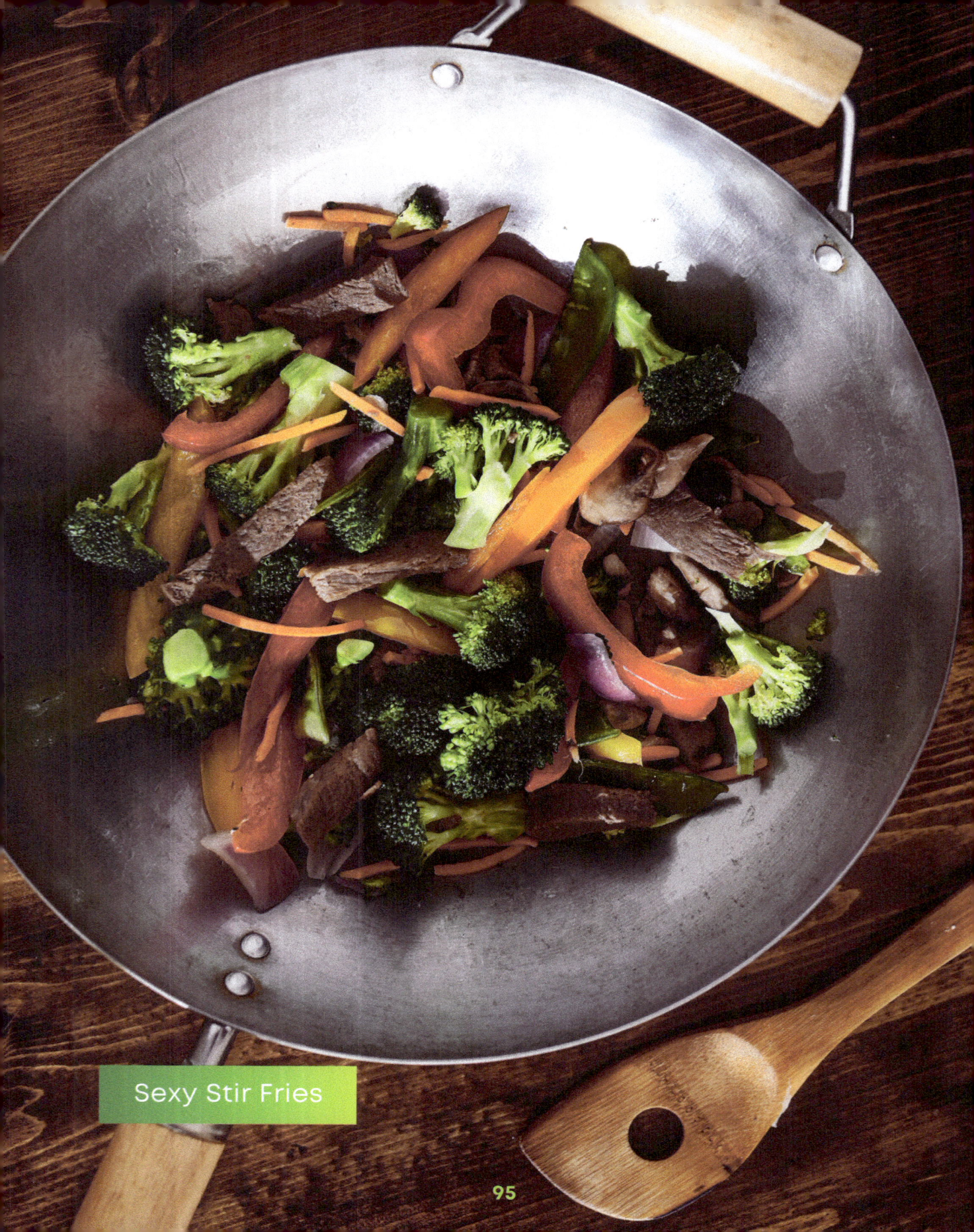

Sexy Stir Fries

Sexy Stir Fries

SERVINGS: 4-6

INGREDIENTS

STIR FRY

1-2 tablespoons peanut/canola/ sunflower/rice bran oil
600g chicken/pork/beef strips
1 cup zucchini, finely sliced or spiralized
1 cup carrots, finely sliced or spiralized
1 cup red onion, finely sliced.
2 cups finely sliced red or wombok cabbage
1 cup finely sliced red capsicum/red pepper
Peanut, chilli, herb bling for crunch
1/2 cup peanuts, crushed and pan toasted
1-2 chopped fresh chillies, or use about half a teaspoon dried
1/2 cup freshly chopped mint/basil/coriander/cilantro

MARINADE

3 tablespoons honey or plum jam
3 tablespoons soy sauce
2 cloves garlic finely crushed
2 tablespoons crushed ginger
1-3 chillies finely chopped
2 drops sesame oil (optional)

METHOD

Remember! Your mission is to keep the sizzle up in your pan...if the pan goes quiet on you, you need to back away from the pan, get some of the pan naked, and then let the pan get back to temperature. HOT HOT HOT Swearword hot.

Put the marinade ingredients over the thin meat strips. Stir to combine.
Heat and grease the pan with the oil. When the pan is smoking hot, add the marinated chicken in a pile on one side of the pan. Please don't spread the meat over the pan, all that will do is smother the heat! Leave the meat in the pile until the first side of the meat that hit the pan, is beautifully brown and sexy and fragrant and sealed. You will need to have a sneaky look underneath one of the pieces using your tongs. Move that meat around by jiggling it with your tongs, but don't stir too much. Don't burn this! Keep checking!
ONLY when that meat is brown underneath do you do a half stir, so that some 'new' meat can hit the base of the pan. Keep doing this, keeping the sizzle high in the pan, until all the meat has been perfectly browned. This way your meat won't stew and you can live happily ever after in the kitchen!

Once all the meat looks heavenly, sticky and brown, start adding the vegetables on the top. You can remove the meat from the pan if your pan is too small for all this action. Stir as much as you like now to get those vegetables hot and wilted right through. Check the seasoning and serve with rice, noodles, or just like that in a bowl with the heavenly peanut bling on top for valuable flavour and crunch!

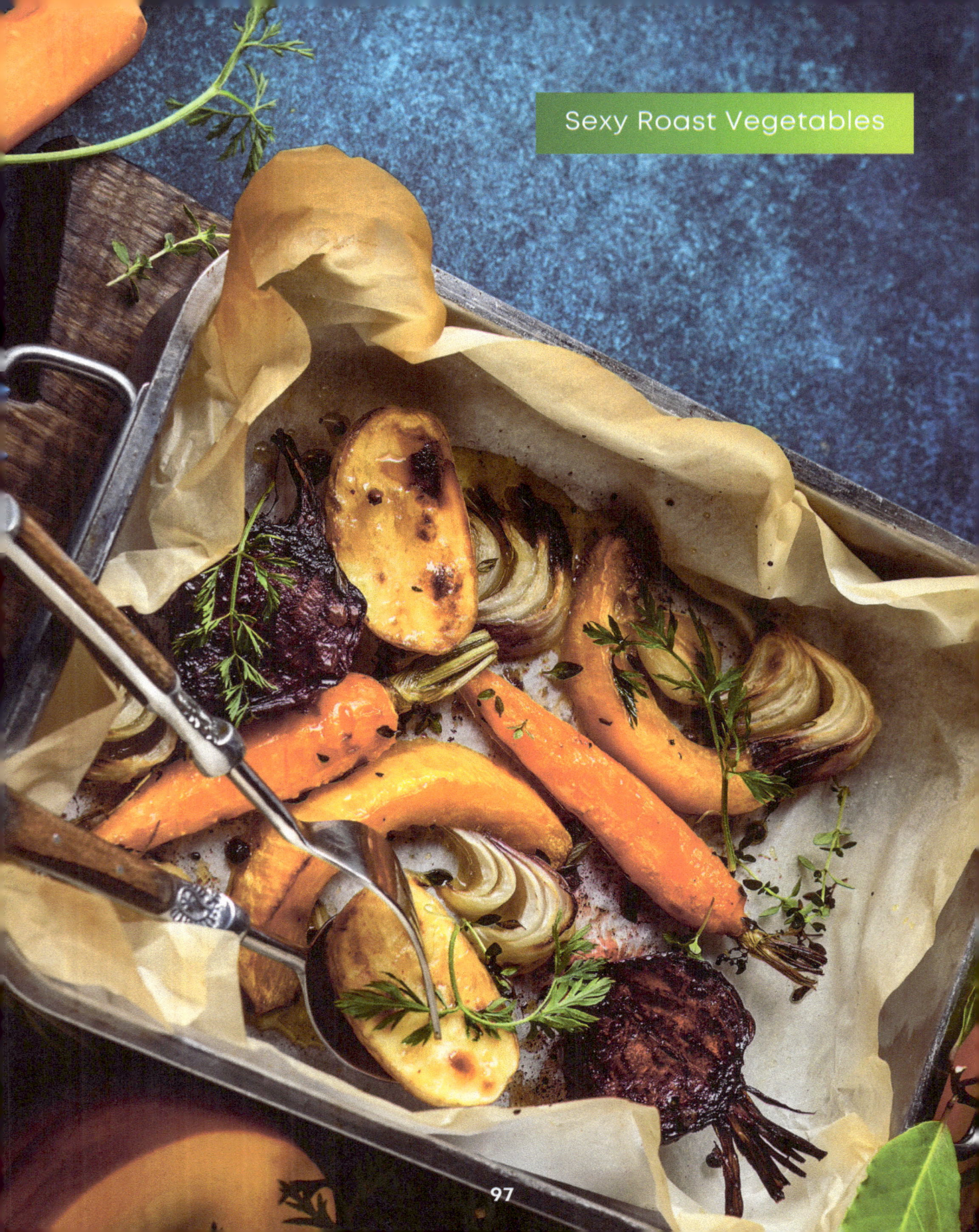

Sexy Roast Vegetables

Sexy Roast Vegetables
(not the pale soggy ones!)

SERVINGS: 2-4

INGREDIENTS

1 cup diced sweet potato
1 cup diced cauliflower
1 cup diced carrot
1 cup diced beetroot
1 cup diced potato
1 cup diced pumpkin

METHOD

CHEF'S NOTE

Always go for colour! Some veggies are better for roasting and some are better for steaming. These veggies are BETTER roasted swear word hot and fast at 220C...this amount of veggies in an oven of 180C will throw SO much steam that they will NEVER go brown.

So, crank the oven up to swear word hot so that we get LOTS of colour in these veggies. When vegetables are roasted they caramelise and give 100% more flavour and personality than when steamed.
I do about a 3cm dice, but you can go bigger or smaller. The larger they are the longer they will take to cook.

Place on a tray and then drizzle with extra virgin olive oil, your choice of spices, salt and pepper. Not too much, these don't need to be drowned or over-spiced, they will be sexy just with a little love.
Cook in a SWEAR WORD HOT oven (220C) for 35 minutes, less if your dice is smaller.
You can use any combination of vegetables that you have available to you.

I always add some green veg after I've roasted the sexy veggies to add some colour and texture.
I steam either beans, snow peas, broccoli or asparagus and then add to the mix.
You can then serve these with a main course, or on their own with either a pea puree or chickpea/butter bean mash to hold the stack together.

Around the World Chicken Breast

SERVINGS: 1

INGREDIENTS

1 chicken breast
2 teaspoons of your favourite spice mix, you can make your own special mix.
It could be curry powder, lemon zest and herbs and garlic,
Oil or water to mix to a paste.
Ras el Hanout, Chinese Five Spice etc

METHOD

Perfect for that quick and easy one pan meal when you just need a healthy lunch.

Cut the chicken breast open lengthways as if you were making schnitzel.
By opening up the breast you help it cook faster. Use the tip of a sharp knife to make some slash cuts, cutting both ways to make a diamond shape. This will allow the flavour to penetrate, and the chicken will cook faster.
Mix your chosen spices with olive oil or water, until you have a thick paste.
Rub the seasoning paste onto the chicken breast on both sides, either using your hands or a brush to get the flavour paste on evenly.
Season with salt and pepper.
Heat and grease a frying pan with vegetable oil, you will only need a little.
Place the chicken into the pan only when it is hot and the chicken sizzles when it hits the pan. Allow to brown perfectly on the first side before turning over and doing the same on the other side.
Reduce the heat and cook through, but take care. This will cook quicker than usual if you have cut in half and done the diamond cuts.
Serve with your favourite veggies or salad.

By changing the spice mixes in your oil or water, you can take your chicken around the world. Try:
GREEK: 1 teaspoon lemon zest, 1 teaspoon lemon juice, 1 teaspoon chopped thyme, basil or other herbs.
FRENCH: 1 tablespoon mustard, 1 teaspoon chopped tarragon or thyme, and zest of a lemon.
THAI: 1 tablespoon Thai curry paste mixed with 2 tablespoons coconut cream and 1 teaspoon fish sauce.
MEXICAN: 1 tablespoon chipotle sauce, 1 tablespoon paprika and a pinch of cinnamon.
SPANISH: 1 tablespoon paprika and 1 teaspoon turmeric with seasoning.
NORTH AFRICAN: 1 tablespoon Ras el Hanout.
You can have so much fun creating flavours. Why not give it a go?

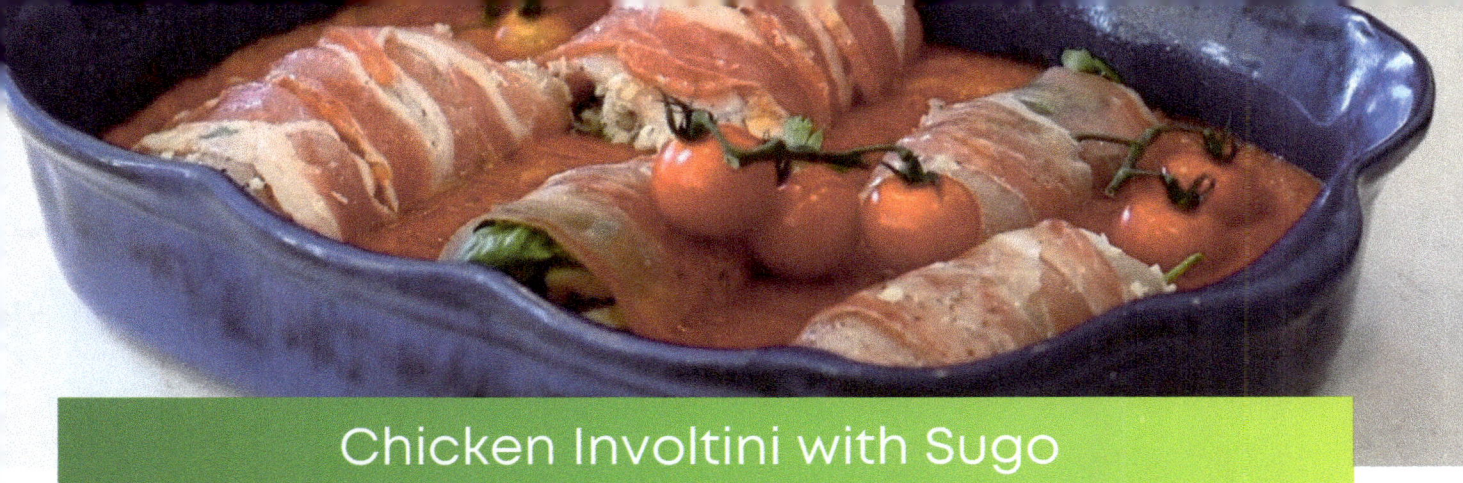

Chicken Involtini with Sugo

SERVINGS: 6-8

INGREDIENTS

INVOLTINI
- 500-600g chicken breast filets
- 12 thinly shaved slices of Prosciutto *or streaky bacon*
- salt and pepper to season
- 80g sliced or grated mozzarella cheese
- 24 fresh basil leaves *or use 2 tablespoons pesto*
- Fresh cherry tomatoes for garnish

SUGO
- 700g jar passata
- 2 cloves garlic, crushed
- 1 teaspoon salt
- large pinch black pepper
- 1 teaspoon dried Italian herbs

METHOD

Take each chicken breast and cut in half lengthways, then open the breast up. Bash with a meat mallet or rolling pin to make sure the breast is tenderised and lovely and thin. Season well with salt and pepper.

Now place 3 slices of the streaky bacon or prosciutto down on your chopping board. Top with the thin chicken breast, sliced or grated cheese, the basil leaves or pesto. You can choose any toppings, mix and match whatever you have such as olives or blue cheese! Carefully roll it up to make a parcel and place in a greased oven dish. Repeat with the remaining chicken breasts.

Make the Quick Sauce by adding all the sauce ingredients together in the passata jar, give it a good shake.

Pour your sauce ingredients around the base of the rolled chicken involtini. Add a few cherry tomatoes around the dish on top of the sauce, but to the side of the chicken.

Drizzle in some lovely, fresh extra virgin olive oil and then bake in a hot oven of approximately 200C for 25-30 minutes until the bacon/prosciutto is brown and delicious, and the chicken has cooked through. Adjust the seasoning of the sauce and then serve.

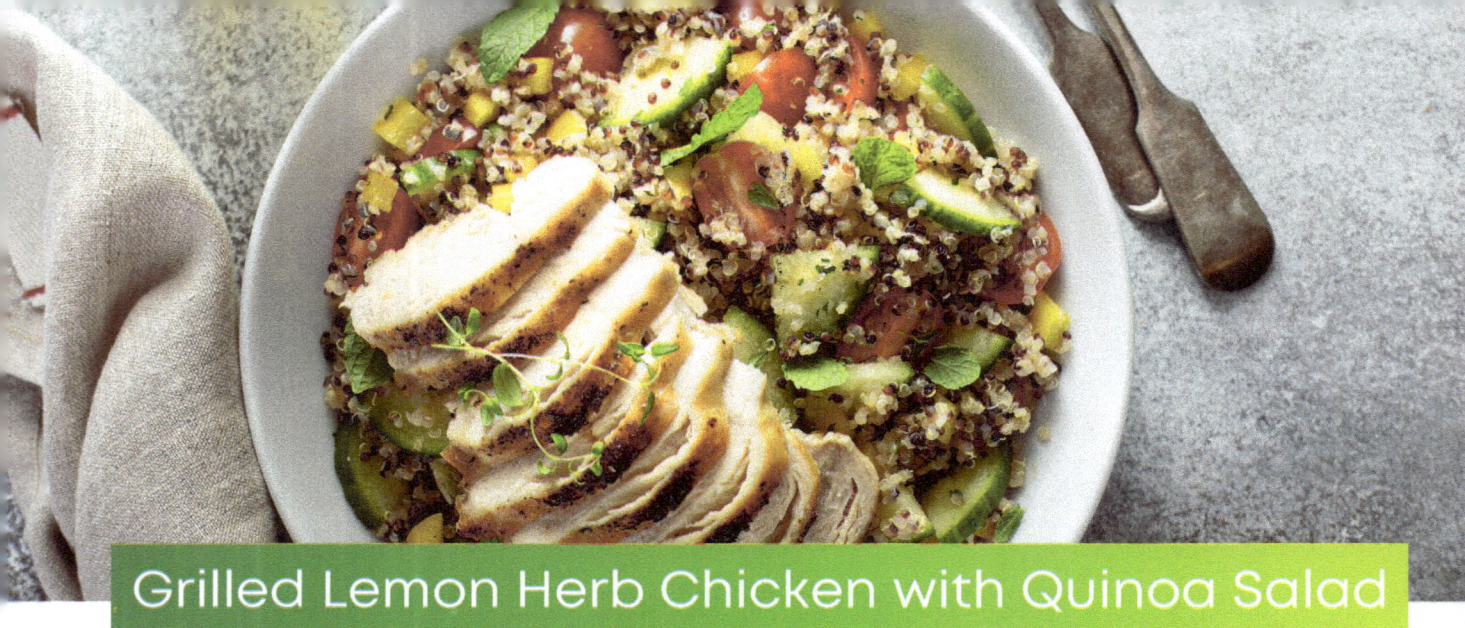

Grilled Lemon Herb Chicken with Quinoa Salad

SERVINGS: 4

INGREDIENTS

4 boneless, skinless chicken breasts
2 lemons, juiced and zested
2 tablespoons olive oil
2 cloves garlic, minced
1 teaspoon dried oregano
1 teaspoon dried thyme
Salt and pepper to taste
1 cup cooked quinoa
1 cup cherry tomatoes, halved
1 cucumber, diced
1/4 cup chopped fresh parsley
1/4 cup crumbled feta cheese (optional)

METHOD

In a bowl, mix the lemon juice, lemon zest, olive oil, garlic, oregano, thyme, salt, and pepper. Marinate the chicken in the mixture for 30 minutes to an hour.

Preheat a grill pan over medium-high heat. You can use the grill element in your oven if you don't have a grill pan.

Grill the chicken for about 6-7 minutes per side or until cooked through.

In a separate bowl, combine the cooked quinoa, cherry tomatoes, cucumber, parsley, and feta cheese (if using). Toss with a drizzle of olive oil and lemon juice.

Serve the grilled chicken alongside the quinoa salad.

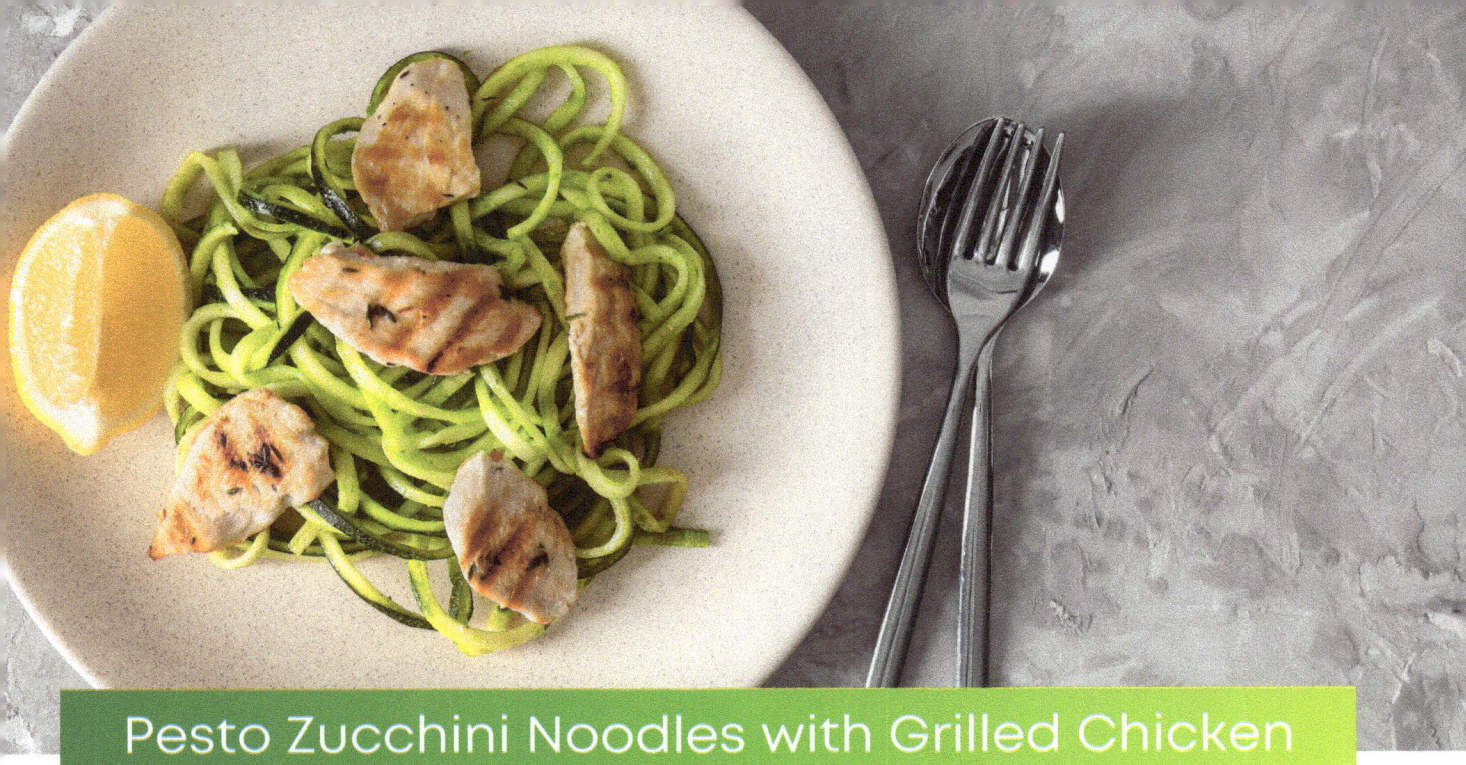

Pesto Zucchini Noodles with Grilled Chicken

SERVINGS: 2

INGREDIENTS

2 large zucchini, spiralized into noodles
(you can use your peeler and make ribbons, or use a spiralizer tool)
2 boneless, skinless chicken breasts, seasoned with salt and pepper
1/4 cup store-bought or homemade pesto
1 tablespoon olive oil
1/4 cup cherry tomatoes, halved
1/4 cup pine nuts (please sniff these and make sure they are fresh)
Fresh basil leaves for garnish
Freshly grated Parmesan or Pecorino

METHOD

Grill the seasoned chicken breasts for about 6-7 minutes per side or until cooked through.
In a large frying pan, heat the olive oil over medium heat.
Add the zucchini noodles and cook for 2-3 minutes until tender but not mushy.

Toss the cooked zucchini noodles with pesto until evenly coated.
Slice the grilled chicken and serve it on top of the pesto zucchini noodles.
Garnish with cherry tomatoes, pine nuts, and fresh basil leaves, and lots of the grated cheese.

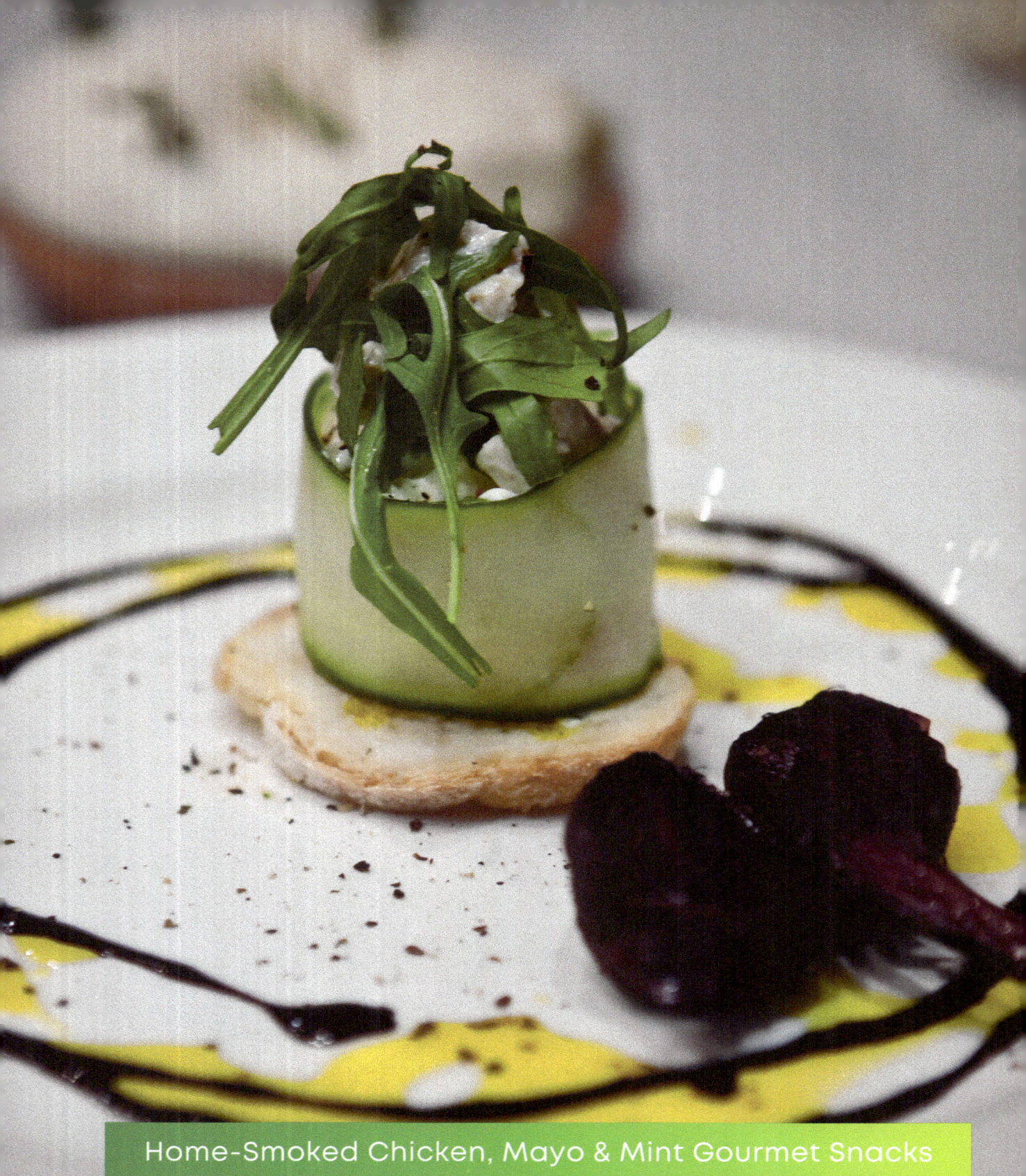

Home-Smoked Chicken, Mayo & Mint Gourmet Snacks

Home-Smoked Chicken, Mayo & Mint Gourmet Snacks

SERVINGS: 2

INGREDIENTS

200g smoked chicken breast fillets, sliced thinly (use smoked salmon if you prefer!)
50ml -100ml fat free yogurt
1 tablespoon freshly chopped mint and/or basil
1 Granny Smith apple, cored and finely sliced
1/2 cup fennel, julienned
1 cup finely chopped broccoli
Lots of ground black pepper
1 teaspoon grainy mustard
1 cucumber, make into ribbons using your peeler
(or slightly roast zucchini ribbons instead)
Slices of roasted sweet potato, lightly coated in your favourite spice…be creative.

METHOD

Roast the sweet potato slices until done in the oven (at 200C) or air fryer.
Place the sweet potato on a large white platter or individual dinner plates.
Mix the chicken, yogurt, fennel, mint, and apple together.
Place a large tablespoon of this in the centre of the sweet potato.

Now use a cucumber or zucchini ribbon to wrap around the filling to create a neat little stack….easy and so gorgeous.

Garnish with lots of ground black pepper and fresh rocket or mustard cress and serve! Drizzle with herbed oil if you're feeling daring.

TO SMOKE THE CHICKEN OR SALMON

Of course you can buy smoked chicken or salad at your local deli or supermarket.

To make yourself, place the chicken or salmon seasoned on a rack. The rack needs to fit into a pot or wok, keeping the chicken or salmon off the base.

Put about 3 tablespoons of tea, lavender or wood sawdust and half a cup plain rice on the base of the pan or wok and then put the lid on and smoke hot and fast for about 12 minutes.
Remove the skin of the salmon and crisp it in the oven.
To get the chicken to smoke faster, simply butterfly and season before smoking.

Quick Durban Chicken Curry

SERVINGS: 4-6

INGREDIENTS

CHICKEN CURRY
- 1-3 tablespoons vegetable oil
- 1 large onion, diced
- 5 cloves garlic, crushed or mashed
- 3 tablespoons ginger, finely mashed
- 2 green chillies, finely chopped (or more if you like this hot)
- 3 tablespoons curry powder
- 1 teaspoon freshly ground cumin
- 1 teaspoon freshly ground coriander/cilantro seed
- 1 teaspoon turmeric powder
- 1 kg chicken thigh, cut into at least three pieces *or go smaller if you like*
- 5 smallish, overripe tomatoes, finely chopped *or use 2 tins*
- 2 small potatoes, dice of about 2cm for a quick cook: *bigger if there is no rush*
- 1 teaspoon salt
- 300ml chicken stock
- 8-10 fresh curry leaves, finely chopped

SAMBALS
- 1 small onion, finely chopped
- 1 large tomato, finely diced
- 1 carrot, peeled and grated
- 3 tablespoons coriander/cilantro, chopped
- 1 green chilli, finely chopped

METHOD

This is really quick to make, but if you possibly can, leave this curry at the end on a very low heat for a further 20 minutes for those flavours to develop. As with any curry, it's even better eaten the day after!

Heat the oil in the pan and add the garlic, chilli, and onion and stir until nicely soft.
Add the spices, taking care not to burn them and allow them to roast off.
Now add the chicken pieces and the salt, and stir to coat. Then let the chicken brown slightly again, taking care not to burn.
Once you have allowed some of the chicken to brown, add the tomatoes and potatoes and the stock. Reduce the heat. Allow to cook through and stir from time to time.
Once the chicken is cooked, the tomatoes have broken down into a delicious thick sauce, and the potatoes are deliciously yellow from the spices, you can add the curry leaves. Season to taste with salt if required. Remember, you must always adjust the seasoning just before serving.

Serve with the sambals.
It's delicious and so quick. This is a Quickie in the Kitchen for sure.

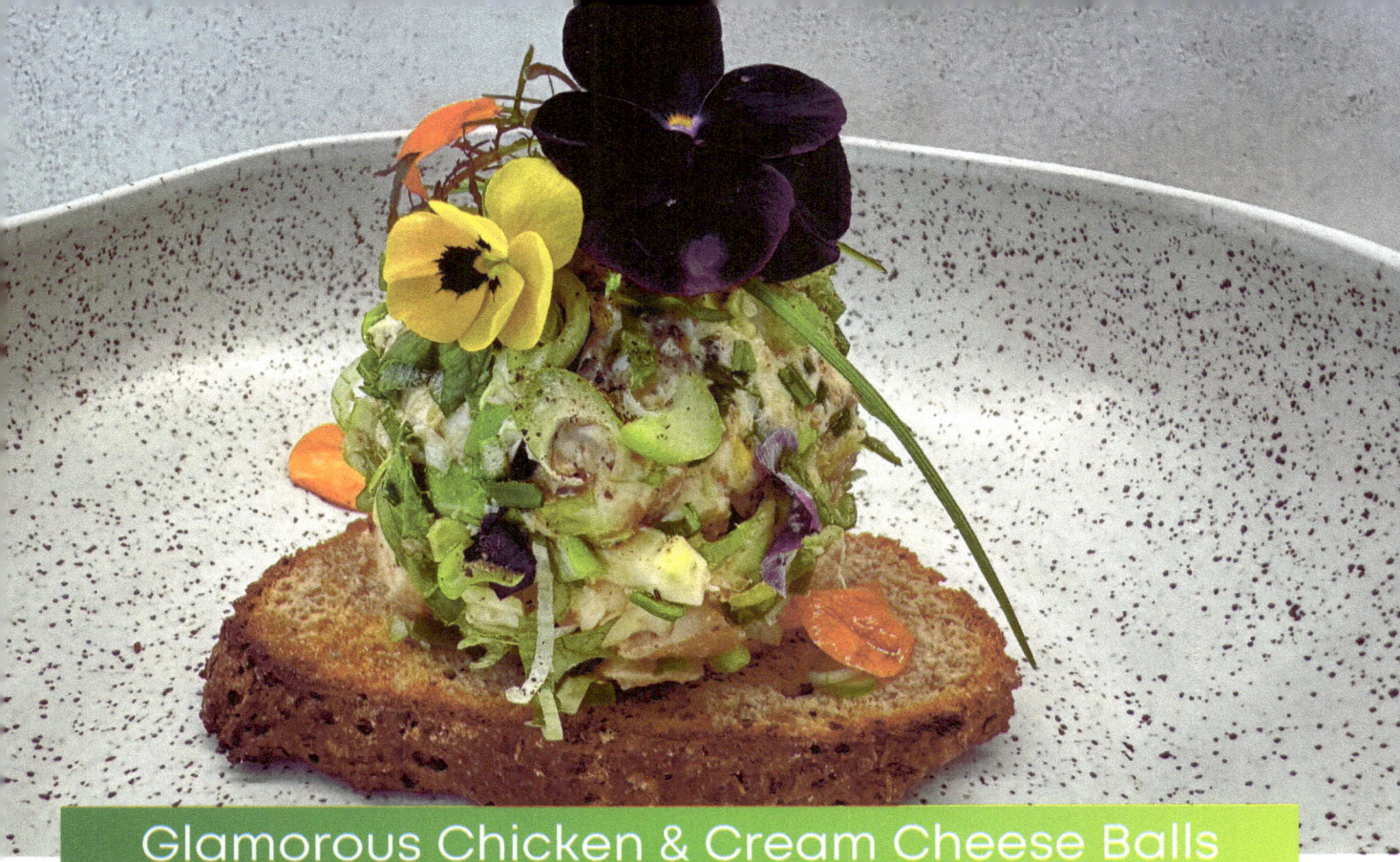

Glamorous Chicken & Cream Cheese Balls

SERVINGS: 4-6

INGREDIENTS

125 g cream cheese, softened
250g chicken or turkey meat, cooked and shredded *(perfect for leftovers)*
zest of one lemon
1 cup chopped broccoli, fennel, cauliflower, green bean, capsicum, cabbage, celery, kale etc.
1 teaspoon mustard
pepper to season
1/2 cup freshly chopped parsley, chives or spring onions to garnish the outside

METHOD

Simply mix the cooked cooled chicken or turkey with the cream cheese, zest, pepper, mustard and veggies.

Stir to bind and then roll into balls.

Drop each ball into and through the chopped parsley or chives and they're ready to serve on a starter platter, as a snack or as a quick and easy dinner!

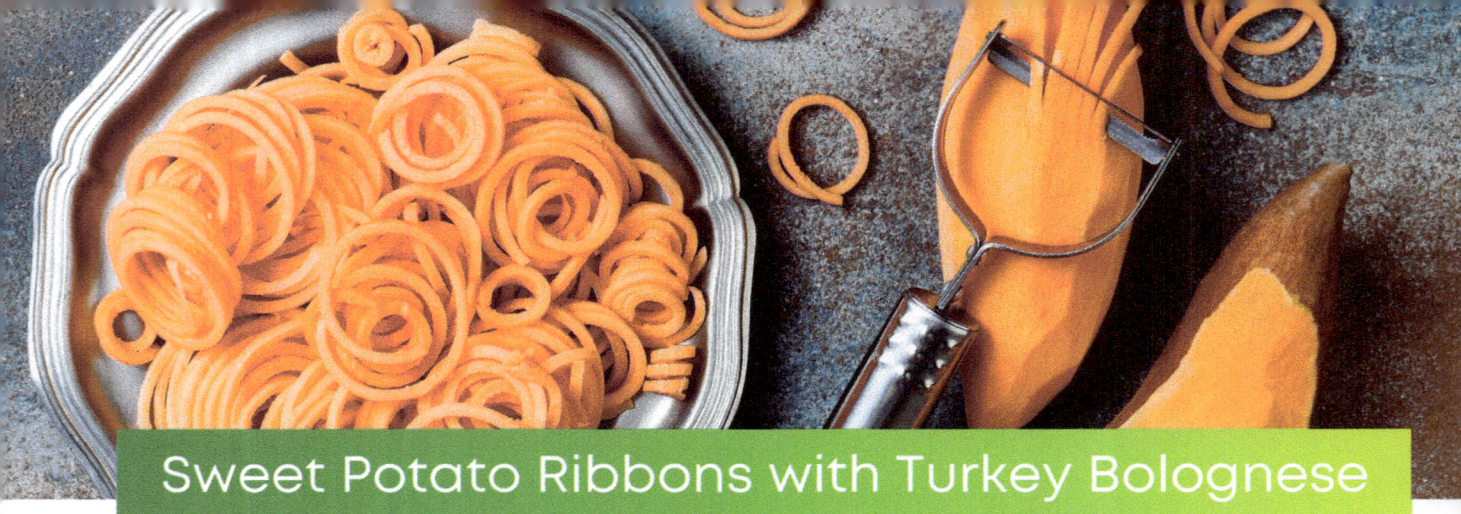

Sweet Potato Ribbons with Turkey Bolognese

SERVINGS: 2-4

INGREDIENTS

400g minced turkey or chicken breast
1 tablespoon olive oil
1 onion, diced
2 cloves garlic, minced
50 ml milk
1ml nutmeg
1 can chopped or crushed tomatoes
1 teaspoon dried basil, or use a handful of fresh leaves
1 teaspoon dried oregano or 1 tablespoon fresh
Salt and pepper to taste
1-2 medium sweet potatoes, washed
Grated Parmesan or Pecorino cheese for garnish (optional)

METHOD

Heat and grease a large frying pan with the olive oil over medium heat. Add the diced onion and garlic, and sauté until translucent. Turn the heat up so the pan is nice and hot so you get a good sizzle when you add the turkey mince.

Cook the turkey or chicken mince until browned. Add the milk and the nutmeg.

Stir in the crushed tomatoes, basil, oregano, salt, and pepper. Let the sauce simmer for about 10-15 minutes.

While your turkey or chicken bolognese is cooking, take your sweet potato and 'peel' it into ribbons using your potato peeler or a spiralizer tool. Either boil these in hot salted water until tender or bake them at 200C or in the air fryer (that's nice and hot) until tender and golden.

Now you can serve your turkey Bolognese sauce over this, and season with some lovely grated Parmesan or Pecorino. Enjoy.

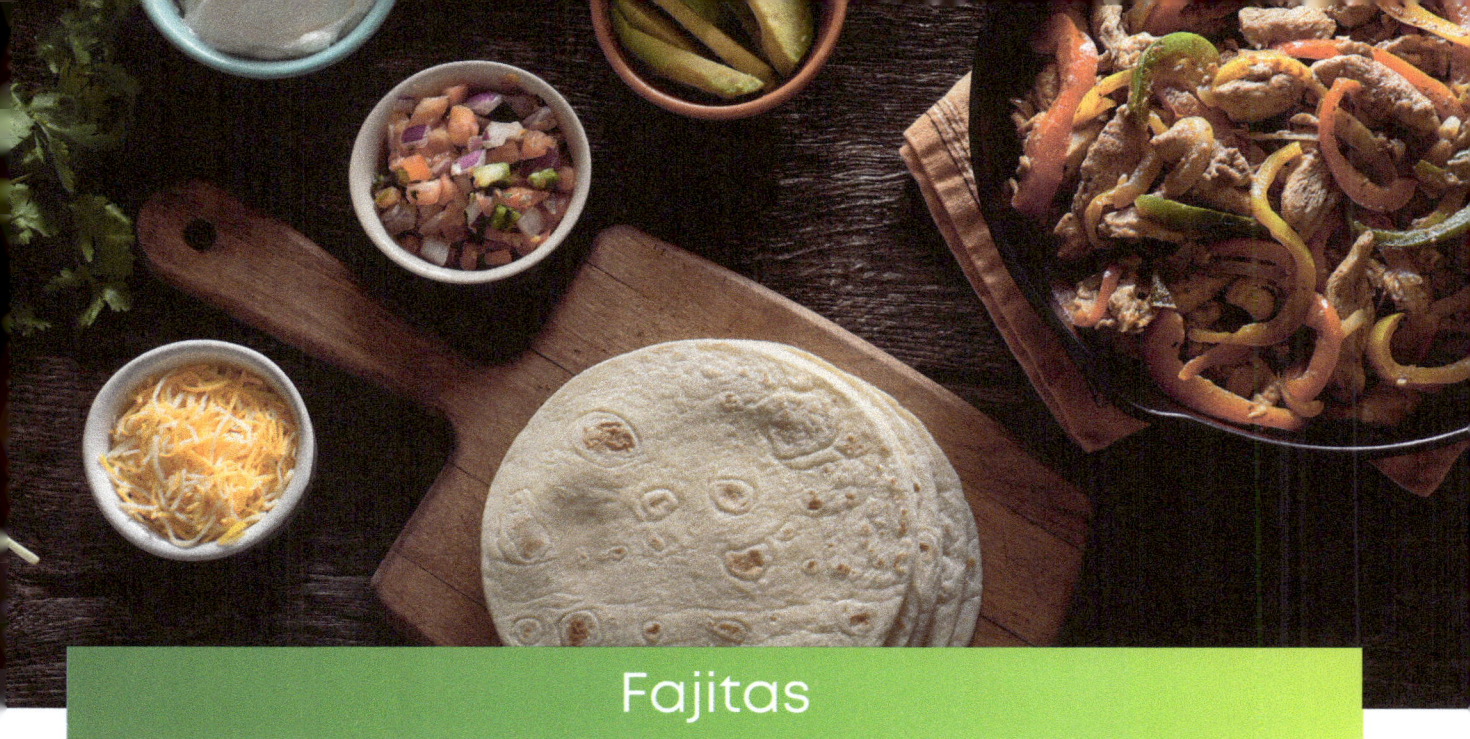

Fajitas

SERVINGS: 1

INGREDIENTS

FILLING	TO SERVE
150 g beef or chicken strips	2 tortillas
1 tablespoons taco or fajita spice	2 tablespoons sour cream
salt and pepper to season	1 tablespoon chopped coriander/cilantro
1 red or brown onion, thinly sliced	1 small chopped chilli
1 large capsicum, thinly sliced	2 tablespoons guacamole

METHOD

Get a frying pan really really hot.

Add about a teaspoon of vegetable oil and allow to sizzle.
Season the strips of beef or chicken with the spices and then add to the pan. Do not stir until the first layer that hit the pan has gone nice and brown, only stir a little to ensure this doesn't burn.

Once cooked add the thinly sliced veggies. I recommend if you are doing this with beef you can keep the beef in a bowl and use the pan to finish cooking the vegetables.
If it's chicken, make sure it's cooked through.
Serve with the tortillas, chopped herbs and the guacamole.
You could also serve with chipotle sauce
Delicious.

Moroccan-Scented Mini Meatloaves
with Cucumber & Cumin Dipping Sauce

SERVINGS: 4

INGREDIENTS

1 teaspoon olive oil
1 large onion, finely chopped
1 clove garlic, finely crushed
3ml turmeric powder
400g lean beef/pork/chicken, minced
Salt and pepper to taste
1/2 teaspoon cumin or Ras el Hanout
Zest of one lemon or lime
1 whole egg beaten, seasoned and mixed with 125ml milk or lightly sour cream (light) to form a custard

METHOD

These are wonderful to make in advance and then cook up as needed!
Fry the onions and the mince in a nice hot pan adding the turmeric and the garlic and the cumin/Ras el Hanout. When browned and fragrant, season to taste and then add the zest and juice of the lemon or lime.
Place the fragrant mince into individual baking dishes and then pour the custard over the mince. Bake for about 12-15 minutes at 180C until just done, these will cook faster in smaller dishes, so beware!

TO WRAP OR GARNISH

Zucchini ribbons slightly roasted (use your blowtorch or griddle pan)

DIPPING SAUCE

1 cup plain fat free yogurt, Pinch of salt and large pinch cumin, 2 tablespoons each cucumber and red onion.

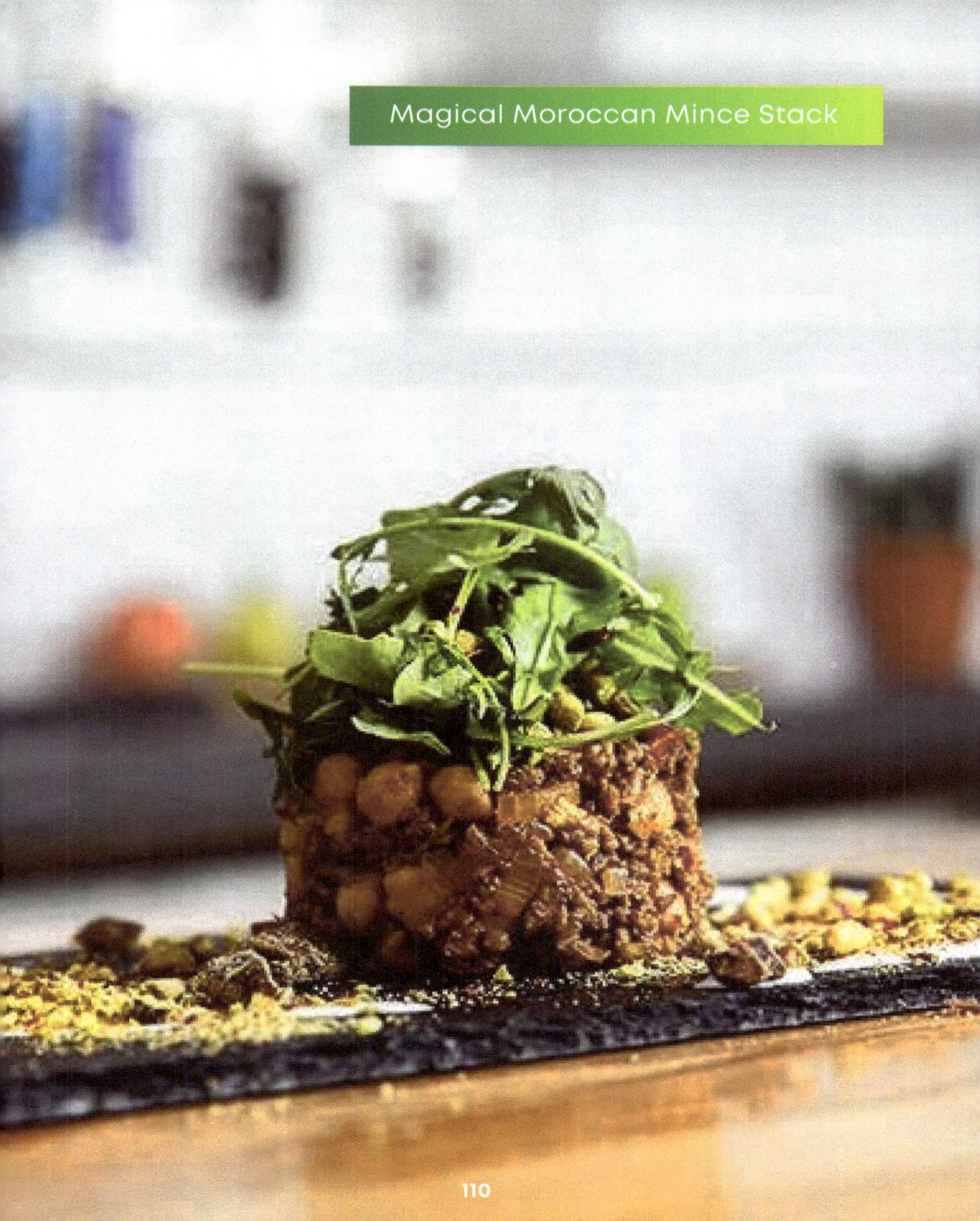

Magical Moroccan Mince Stack

Magical Moroccan Mince Stack
with Pistachio & Date Gravel

SERVINGS: 4-6

INGREDIENTS

MOROCCAN MINCE STACK

2 squirts of canola or rice bran cooking spray

800g lean beef mince
(fluff this up with your hands so it's nice, loose, fluffy & not in 1 big block)

1 large onion, finely diced

1 clove garlic, crushed (optional)

1 tablespoon Ras el Hanout
(you can make your own using 1 teaspoon cumin powder, 1/2 teaspoon cardamom powder and 1/2 teaspoon coriander/cilantro powder)

1 teaspoon turmeric

1/2 cup finely diced fennel
or you could use grated carrot/zucchini

1 tin chickpeas, drained & rinsed

1 cup or tin chopped tomatoes

2 tablespoons tomato paste or passata

1 vegetable or beef stock cube crumbled to a powder

Salt & pepper to season

About 1 teaspoon of lemon zest

PISTACHIO & DATE GRAVEL

1-2 tablespoons pistachios, bashed *or chopped to a nice coarse gravel*

2 tablespoons finely chopped dates

Dried rose petals, but if you don't have that: *grate in some lemon zest (1/2 teaspoon) and 1 tablespoon finely chopped parsley or coriander/cilantro for colour*

METHOD

Grease a large pan with the oil spray and heat the pan until it's just about smoking hot. The mince MUST sizzle when it hits the pan.

Now add the mince that you have broken up in the packaging or a bowl so it is loose and fluffy already. Put the mince into the pan. IT SHOULD SIZZLE nice and loud and sexy.

DO NOT STIR, I know you are worried about this burning and you are also worried about lumps, but let the mince brown and seal on the first side you put down FIRST and let the pan heat up again and THEN you can stir ever so slightly just to get some more mince onto the base of the pan. My favourite mince 'fluffer' is one of those cheap plastic-coated whisks you get at the supermarket that only have about 4 loops. If you don't have one of those use a strong plastic spoon or egg flip to break down the mince.

Once the mince is brown and fragrant and sexy ALL BY ITSELF, then and only then, do you add the finely chopped onion and garlic. There should be a good amount of fat rendered out of the mince during your amazing sizzling at a nice high heat.

You can stir as much as you like now by the way. That mince is SEALED off!

Now add the spices, stock powder and seasoning and stir through. Amazing colour isn't it. Finally, add the chopped tomatoes and passata and the chickpeas and you're practically done. Turn down the heat and let that all cook through and then add the lemon zest and it's ready to serve. This way of cooking will not only save you time, BUT it will add valuable flavour and vibrant personality to your otherwise boring mince. I love to get creative with my mince and change the spices thus changing the flavour. I pack mine into a food stacker and serve it with a yogurt swirl, the pistachio and date gravel, and just a twist of fresh, peppery rocket leaves.

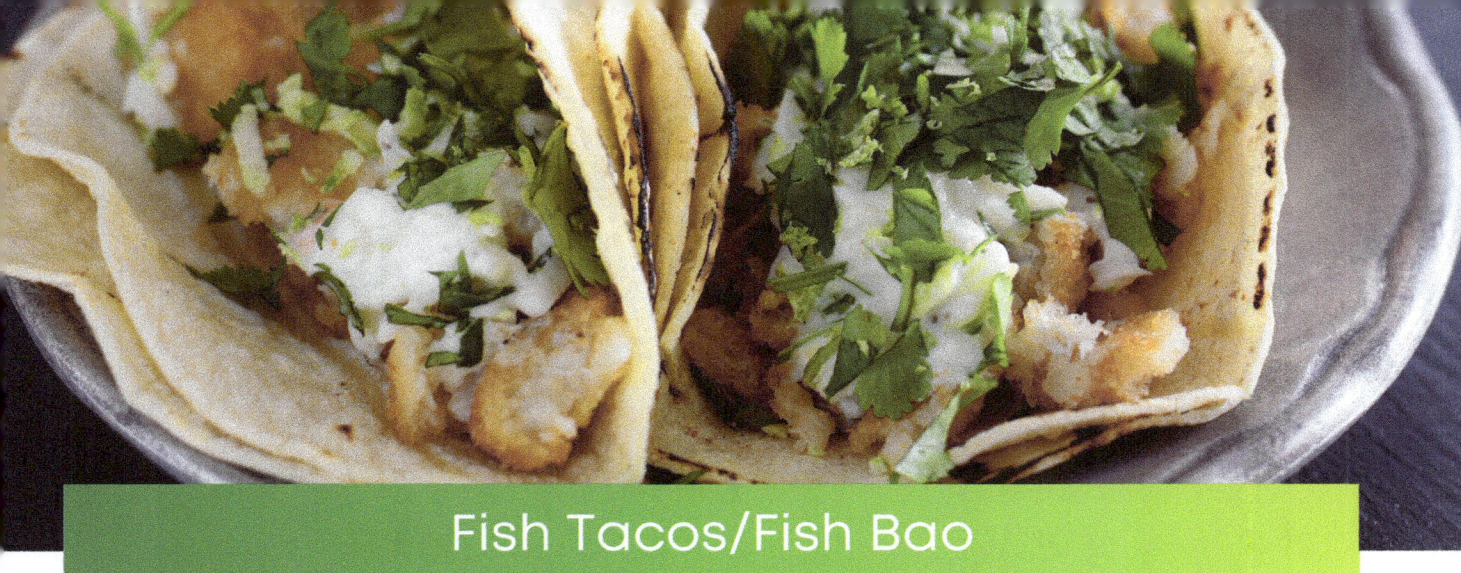

Fish Tacos/Fish Bao

SERVINGS: 1

INGREDIENTS

FISH & BAO
100g fresh fish, skin on
salt and pepper or taco spice to season
4-8 mini tortilla wrappers or bao buns
4 tablespoons chopped kale
4 tablespoons grated carrot
1 teaspoon chopped coriander/cilantro
1 chopped chilli
1 small chopped red onion
4 tablespoons chopped spinach or lettuce

DRESSING
4 tablespoon Kewpie or Mayo
4 tablespoons water
3 drops sesame oil
1 teaspoon sesame seeds

METHOD

Season the fish pieces well and then place the fish, skin side up on a greased baking tray or air fryer.

Bake at 220C for 8 minutes, then remove from the oven and use your tongs to remove the fish skin. It will release quite easily now that the fish is nearly cooked.
Put the skin on the tray to the side and cook for a further 6 minutes or until the skin is crisp and the fish is cooked through.

Now cut into large chunks and serve with the tortilla wrapper or bao buns.
Fill with the gorgeous veggies.
Dress with the sexy dressing and enjoy.
If you're off the carbs, simply serve as a bowl of goodness.

Thai Fish Cakes

SERVINGS: 6-8

INGREDIENTS

FISH CAKES

1 garlic clove, smashed
3 lime leaves, finely chopped
2 tablespoons coarsely chopped fresh coriander/cilantro *root or leaves*
1 tablespoon fish sauce
500g firm white fish fillets, coarsely chopped
3 teaspoons Thai curry paste
Pinch of salt
3-5 snake or green beans, thinly sliced
Peanut oil or coconut oil

DIPPING SAUCE

1/4 cup white sugar
1/4 cup fresh lime juice
1 tablespoon fish sauce
1 finely chopped shallot
1/4 cucumber, deseeded, finely chopped
1 small fresh red Birdseye chilli, deseeded, thinly sliced
Thai lime leaves, chopped into a dust

METHOD

Place the cubed fish and garlic in the bowl of a food processor and process until finely chopped. Add the lime leaves, coriander/cilantro, fish sauce, curry paste and salt, and process until just combined. Transfer fish mixture to a bowl. Add the beans and stir to combine.

Divide the fish mixture into equal portions. The best way to shape these is using wet hands to form into thick patties. Place on a plate on some greaseproof paper or chopping board. Heat oil in a large frying pan until really hot. Cook patties on each side until light brown and cooked through.

Transfer to a plate lined with paper towel. Repeat with the remaining patties, reheating pan between batches.

Combine the dipping sauce ingredients in a small saucepan over medium heat. Cook, stirring, for 5 minutes or until sugar dissolves.

Remove from heat. Add the cucumber, shallot and chilli and stir to combine.

Serve hot or cold! These fabulous fish cakes can be made the day in advance and then cooked closer to the time! Enjoy!

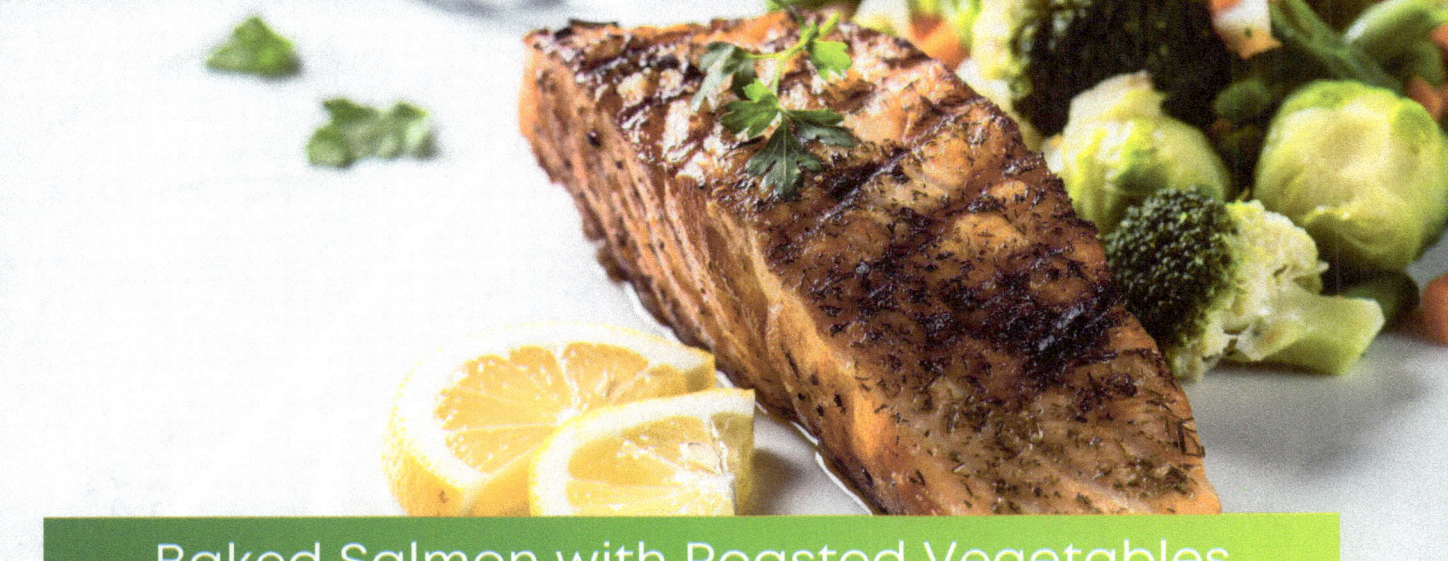

Baked Salmon with Roasted Vegetables

SERVINGS: 4

INGREDIENTS

4 salmon fillets, about 150g each
2 tablespoons olive oil
1 teaspoon paprika
1/2 teaspoon garlic powder
Salt and pepper to taste
2 cups broccoli florets
2 cups cherry tomatoes
1 red capsicum/pepper, sliced
1 yellow capsicum/pepper, sliced
1 tablespoon balsamic vinegar

METHOD

Preheat the oven to about 200C. It really does need to be nice and hot.

Line a baking sheet with baking paper and then place the salmon fillets on the baking sheet. Drizzle with olive oil and sprinkle with paprika, garlic powder, salt, and pepper.

In a separate bowl, toss the broccoli, cherry tomatoes, and bell peppers with olive oil, salt, and pepper. Spread the vegetables around the salmon on the baking sheet. Drizzle with balsamic vinegar.

Bake in the preheated oven for about 15-20 minutes, or until the salmon is cooked through and the vegetables are tender and baked golden.
Delicious!

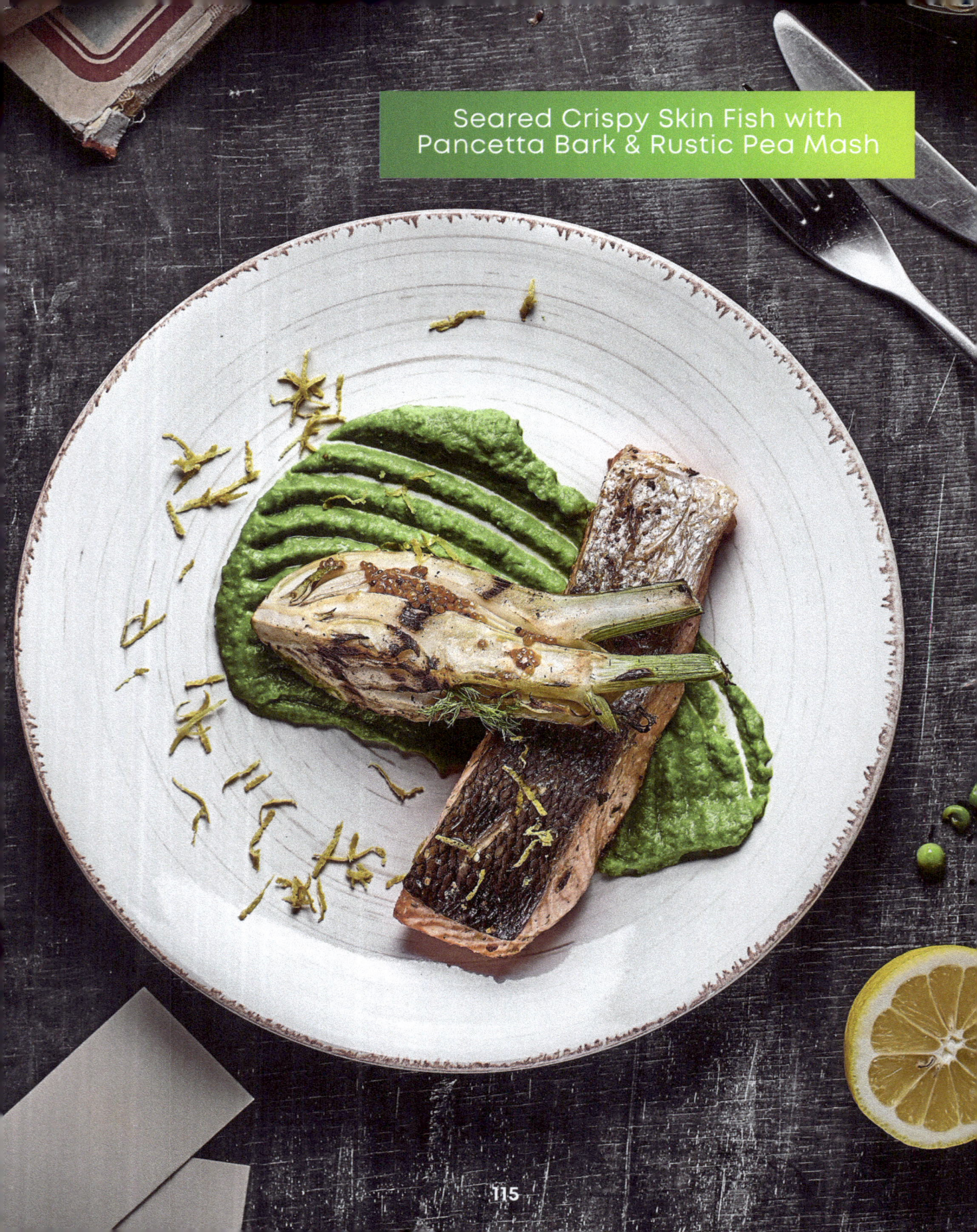

Seared Crispy Skin Fish with Pancetta Bark & Rustic Pea Mash

Seared Crispy Skin Fish
with Pancetta Bark & Rustic Pea Mash

SERVINGS: 4-6

INGREDIENTS

FISH & PANCETTA BARK

600-800g fish, skin on
Salt and pepper to season
Half lemon or lime per serving
4-6 strips Pancetta
placed on a roasting tray and then baked until crispy in a hot oven of 200C

RUSTIC PEA PURÉE

2 cups frozen peas
1 onion, finely chopped
1 clove garlic minced
150-250ml chicken or vegetable stock
(depending on thickness required… please adjust)
20g butter
80-150ml cream

METHOD

This is my favourite recipe for when I am entertaining because it is practically stress free! A beautiful piece of fish or salmon needs little masking and if cooked perfectly, will simply shine.

Firstly, get your pan or BBQ SWEAR WORD HOT and grease with about 5 ml vegetable or rice bran oil. You can also do this in your air fryer. This will make sure that the fish doesn't stick. When the pan is hot, place the fish **skin side up**, and use your tongs to make sure it doesn't stick…I just give the piece a little wiggle to make sure it hasn't stuck but will create a sexy crust of flavour and colour. When the first side is brown (simply look underneath and lift with your tongs) turn it over to cook the skin side too. After about a minute or two you should be able to remove the skin using the tongs.
Don't stress if it breaks or you have to strip-peel it off, it is all part of the rustic glamour of this dish! Place the skin aside and then turn the now skin-free side down to brown it off. When the fish is cooked (check by placing a fork or knife in the centre of the thickest part and if it flakes when you twist it is done!), remove it from the pan. Lower the heat and fry the skin nice and hot (but not so hot that it burns in a flash) as this will dry and crisp up the skin
NEVER serve soggy fish skin…it is just not glamorous and can be easily crisped up by just allowing it some alone time in the pan.
Serve with this amazingly versatile pea puree! Don't like peas? Use butterbeans (drained out of a tin) instead!

RUSTIC PEA PURÉE

Place all the ingredients into a medium saucepan and boil over a medium heat for about 15 minutes. Remove from the heat and blend to a smooth puree with a stick blender or manual masher. Adjust the seasoning and thickness and then serve.

Giant Tiger Prawns with Peri Peri

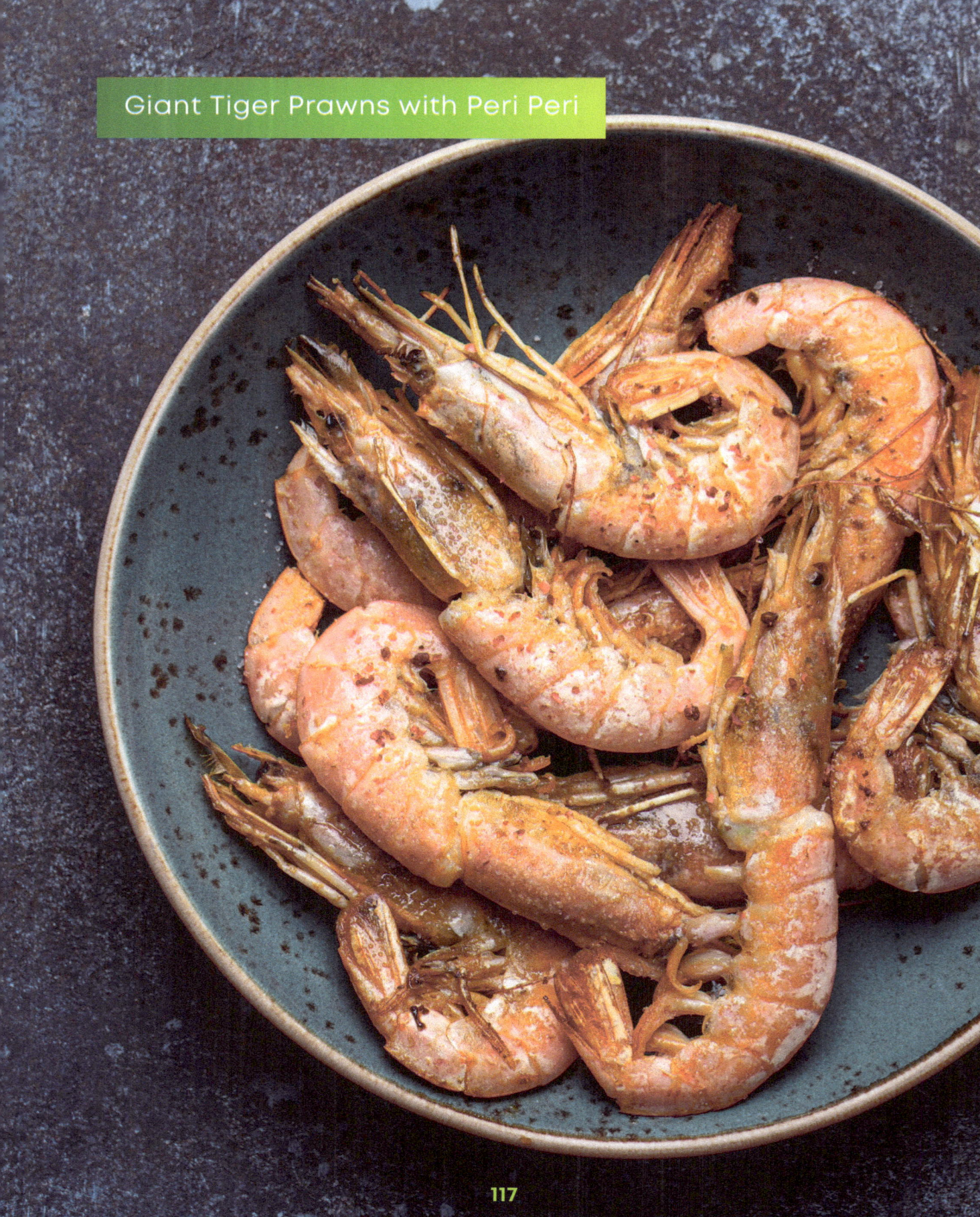

Giant Tiger Prawns with Peri Peri

SERVINGS: 2-4

INGREDIENTS

1kg giant tiger prawns
2 onions, finely chopped
6 cloves garlic, minced
10 birds eye chillies
1 cup lemon juice
zest of one lemon
1 cup olive oil
1 teaspoon salt
1 teaspoon sugar
2 tablespoons hot or sweet paprika
Lemons halves to serve

METHOD

Clean and devein the prawns by cutting down the back of the prawn with a good pair of kitchen scissors and removing the vein. Keep the shell on. You can cut almost right through the prawn to butterfly them OR just leave them whole.

Pop all the other ingredients into a food processor and whizz until it forms a thick fragrant paste, or you can chop it the good old fashioned way. Now use this sauce to marinate your prawns.

To cook the prawns in their lovely sauce, simply heat your greased pan or outside on the BBQ or coal fire to a good but medium heat and then place the prawns, flesh side down, and get them nicely browned and sealed off before turning over and browning the shell. They don't take long so please don't overcook!

Serve with lemon halves, browned in a pan until juicy and delicious.

"Cooking is a philosophy; it's not a recipe."
— Marco Pierre White

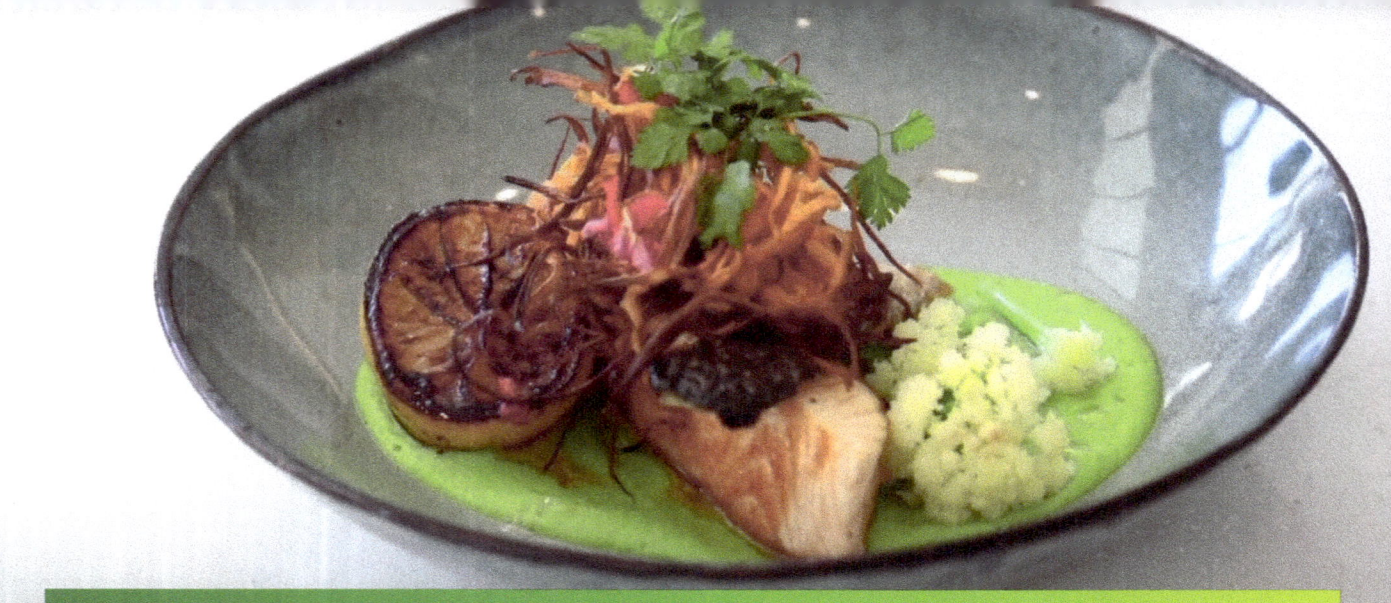

Tea Smoked Crispy Skin Salmon

SERVINGS: YOU DECIDE

INGREDIENTS

Cooking oil or spray (not olive)
80-100g salmon per person, with skin
salt and pepper to season
1/2 cup black or rooibos tea leaves
1/2 cup rice, any kind
2-3 star anise, cardamom or cinnamon (you choose)

METHOD

CHEF'S NOTE:
You will need a pot that can fit a cake rack or colander inside, with a tight-fitting lid
OR a deep frying pan with lid and a cake rack that can fit inside
You MUST have a close-fitting lid.

Grease the colander or rack with the oil or cooking spray.
Place the seasoned fish pieces skin side up on the rack. Place the rice, tea and spices in the pan and then put the fish on the rack on top. Close with a lid. Place on full heat. When you see smoke, THEN time for 15 minutes. The fish will cook when the hot smoke starts to circulate.

When 15 minutes is done, take the pot/pan OUTSIDE and to remove the lid.
Remove the skin using tongs, and place on a greased baking tray.
Pop under the preheated grill or in a hot oven at 200C until the skin is crispy and perfect.
Serve with pea puree, caramelised lemon and the crispy skin.
Perfect and so quick and easy and healthy.

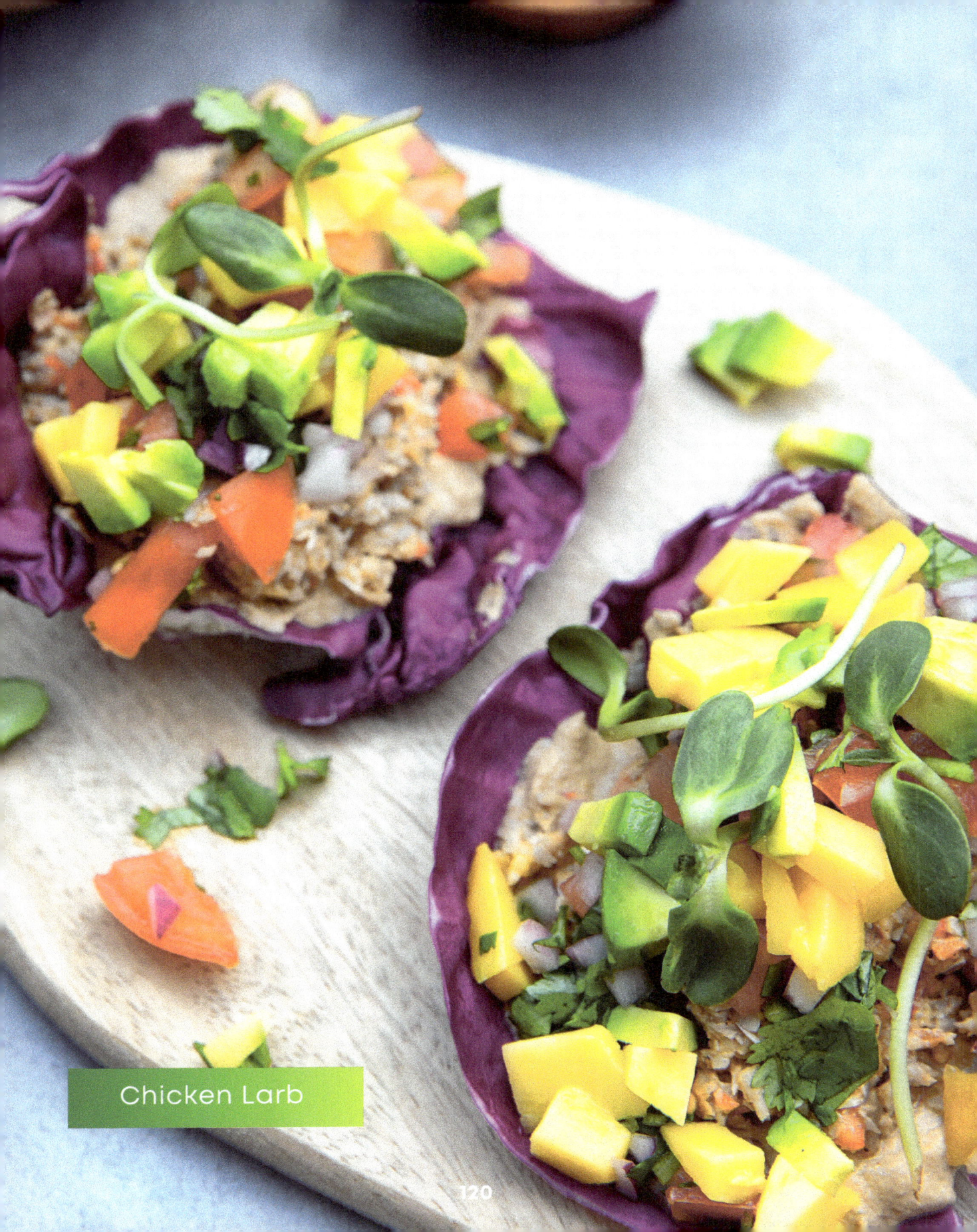

Chicken Larb

Chicken Larb

SERVINGS: 6-8

INGREDIENTS

LARB

- 400-600g chicken mince
- 1 tablespoon vegetable oil
- 1 shallot, finely chopped
- 2 cloves garlic, minced
- 1 teaspoon ginger, minced
- 1-2 Thai chillies, finely chopped (adjust to taste)
- 1/4 cup chopped fresh herbs (a combination of mint, cilantro/coriander, and Thai basil)
- 2 green onions, chopped
- 1/4 cup toasted rice powder (grind dry rice in a blender or spice grinder)
- Salt, to taste

DRESSING

- 3 tablespoons fish sauce
- 2 tablespoons lime juice
- 1 tablespoon soy sauce
- 1 teaspoon brown sugar/palm sugar/maple

FOR SERVING

- Lettuce leaves or cabbage leaves
- Sliced cucumber
- Sliced red onion
- Extra lime wedges

METHOD

Heat the vegetable oil in a pan over medium heat. Add the chopped shallot, garlic, and ginger. Sauté until fragrant. Add the ground chicken mince to the pan and break it up into small pieces with a spatula. Cook until the chicken is cooked through and no longer pink.

While the chicken is cooking, prepare the dressing. In a bowl, mix together the fish sauce, lime juice, soy sauce, and sugar until the sugar is dissolved.

Once the chicken is cooked, add the chopped Thai chillies and stir-fry for another minute.

Remove the pan from the heat and add the chopped fresh herbs, green onions, and toasted rice powder to the chicken. Mix well.

Pour the dressing over the chicken mixture and toss everything together until well combined.

Taste and adjust the seasoning, adding salt or more fish sauce if needed.

So easy! To serve, arrange lettuce leaves or cabbage leaves on a plate. Spoon the chicken larb onto the leaves, it's like an edible plate...

Garnish the larb with sliced cucumber, sliced red onion, and extra herbs.

Serve the chicken larb with lime wedges on the side.

You can enjoy the chicken larb by wrapping spoonfuls of it in the lettuce leaves or cabbage leaves, creating little bundles of deliciousness.

Remember that the spiciness level can be adjusted by adding or reducing the amount of Thai chillies. This recipe is quite customizable, so feel free to experiment with the ingredients and quantities to suit your taste preferences.

Treats, Snacks & Desserty Treats

It's time for a delcious treat.

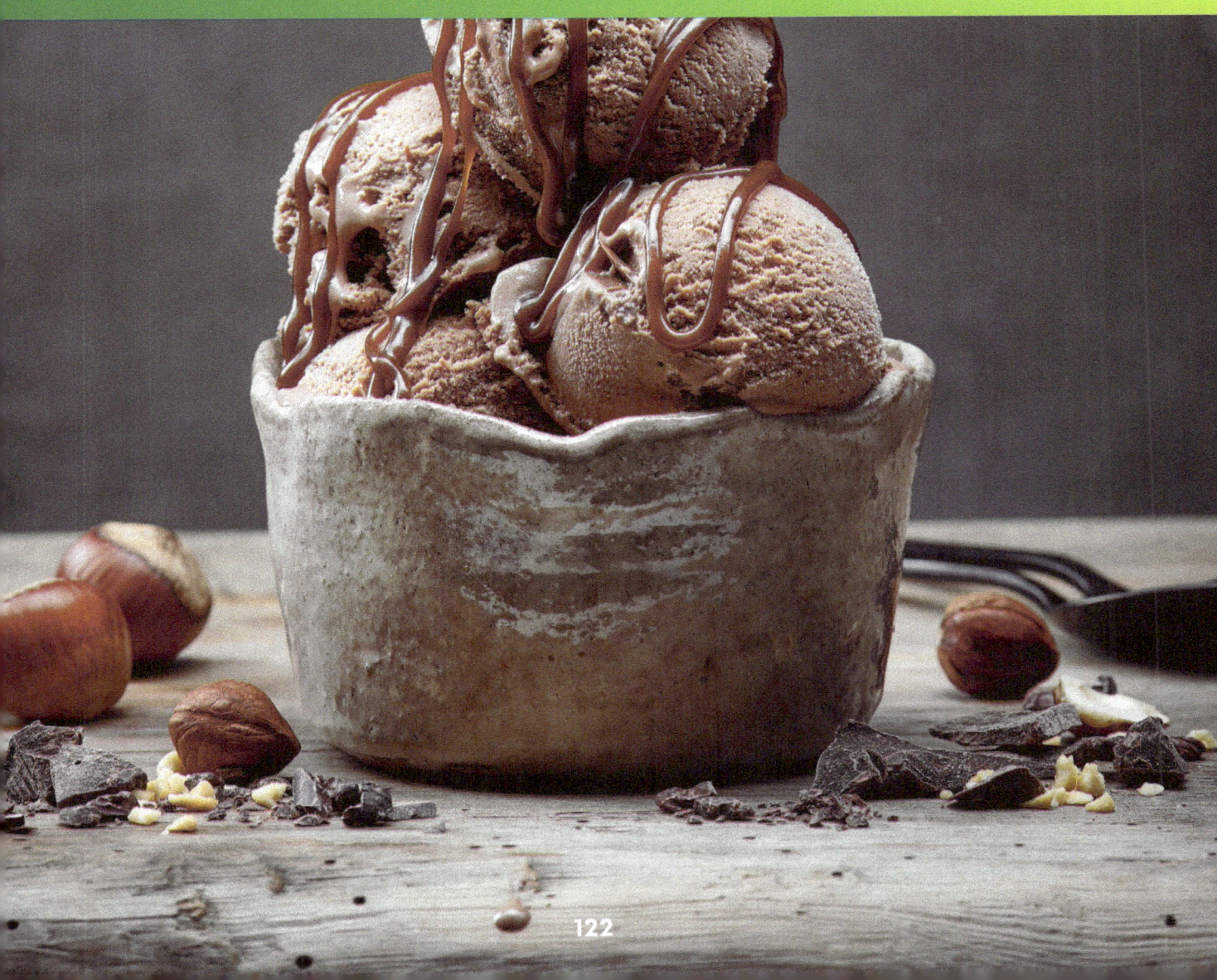

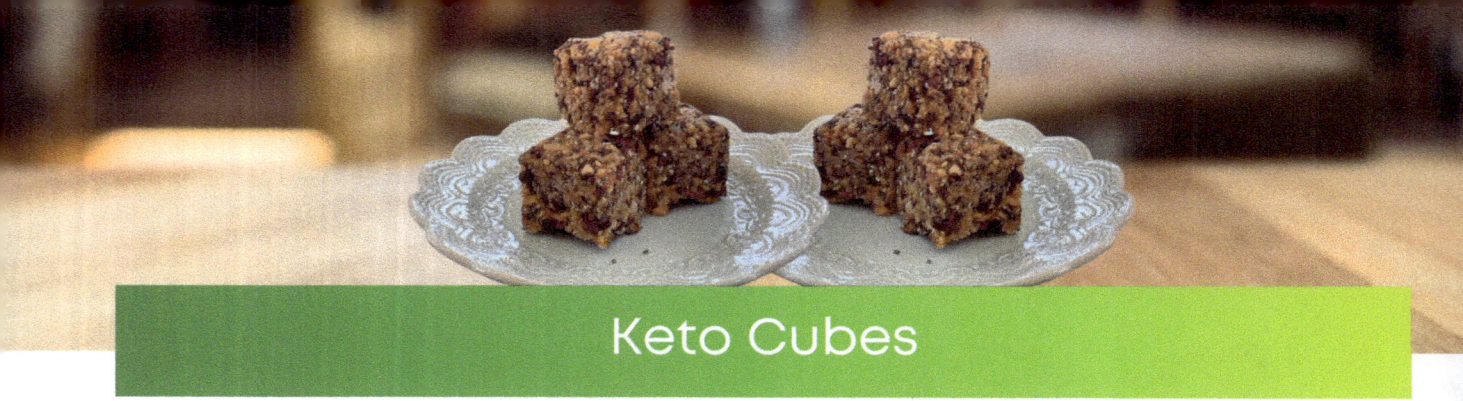

Keto Cubes

SERVINGS: 36 CUBES

INGREDIENTS

1 cup chopped whole nuts
(choose from almond, macadamia, Brazil or hazel, any of these will do.
I pop mine in the food processor to blitz them into a nut gravel so they toast faster)
1 cup shredded or desiccated coconut
1 cup dates, chopped or blended in processor (or use 1/4 cup powdered sweetener if you prefer)
1 cup chia seeds, black or white
1 cup peanut butter, I used crunchy organic
1/2 cup cocoa nibs
1/2 cup 70-90% dark chocolate, chopped or blended in processor
5ml vanilla extract
1/2 cup water
1 cup protein/whey powder. You could use an almond meal instead.

METHOD

CHEFS NOTE

So when you need a really healthy alternative to sugar and naughty chocolate, you will LOVE my quick and easy and extremely nutritious cubes of pleasure. Bursting with health-promoting ingredients, with no baking required, these will be a handy little pick me up for those days when you just 'need a little something'! This recipe is quite big, and very versatile, and it gives me, my boys and my hubbie fabulous little treats to grab out of the freezer on the way out the door. You can store these in the pantry on the shelf, but I make them in my silicone ice cube trays and freeze them so that they are there for weeks or months (perfect if you have a smaller family than mine!). Feel free to follow my versatile options and make these YOUR own favourite treat.

Place the chopped/blended nut gravel and coconut into a frying pan on high heat. Cook for 2-3 minutes stirring to toast them until they are nice and brown and deliciously fragrant. Don't burn.
Place this and the remaining ingredients into your stand mixer bowl with the whisk and mix for about a minute until it forms a sticky, wet crumb.
Use a spoon over the bowl to fill and then pack (using the back of the spoon) the ice cube trays.
Place the trays on a flat surface and then pack tight with the palm of your hand, the chia and water and protein powder will start to set and keep these gorgeous treats together.
Pop in the fridge or freezer, covered, and then enjoy every time you need a treat.

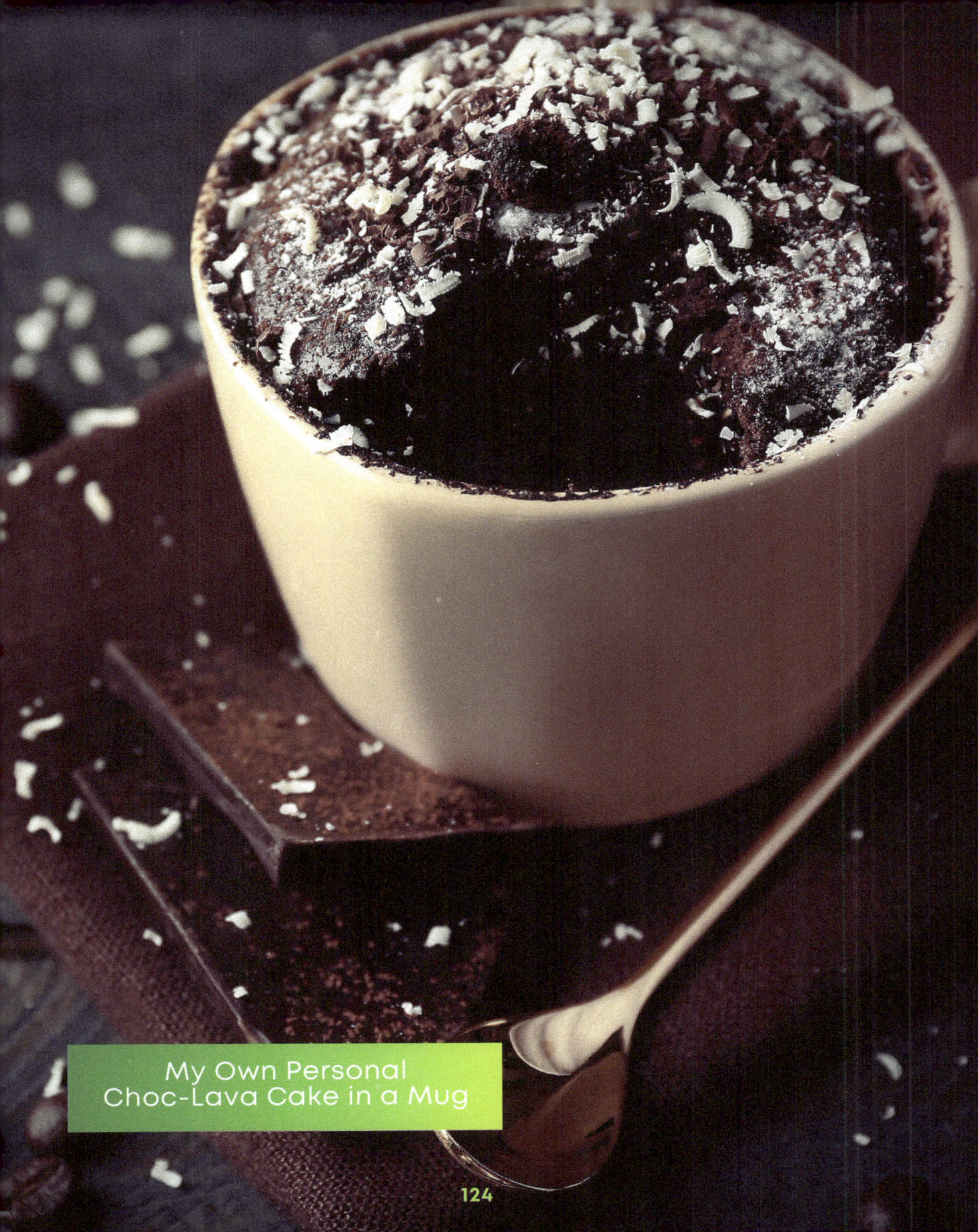

My Own Personal Choc-Lava Cake in a Mug

My Own Personal Choc-Lava Cake in a Mug

SERVINGS: 2

INGREDIENTS

Eat one now, keep the one in the freezer for later

1 egg
1/2 teaspoon baking powder
2 tablespoons almond meal/plain flour
2 tablespoons coconut flour/plain flour
2 tablespoons cocoa powder
2 tablespoons vegetable oil or melted butter
2 tablespoons sweetener or 2 tablespoons sugar
2 tablespoons dark chocolate chips
4 tablespoons milk
1 pinch salt
1 teaspoon vanilla extract or paste

METHOD

Easiest treat ever.

Mix all the ingredients together to make a thick batter.

Grease two coffee mugs and then divide the beautiful batter between them.

Cook one at a time in the microwave for 50 seconds until just done, but slightly gooey in the middle is best. You can cook both, or you can keep one in the freezer for later.

The chocolate buttons should melt and provide a decadent bit of oozy chocolate.

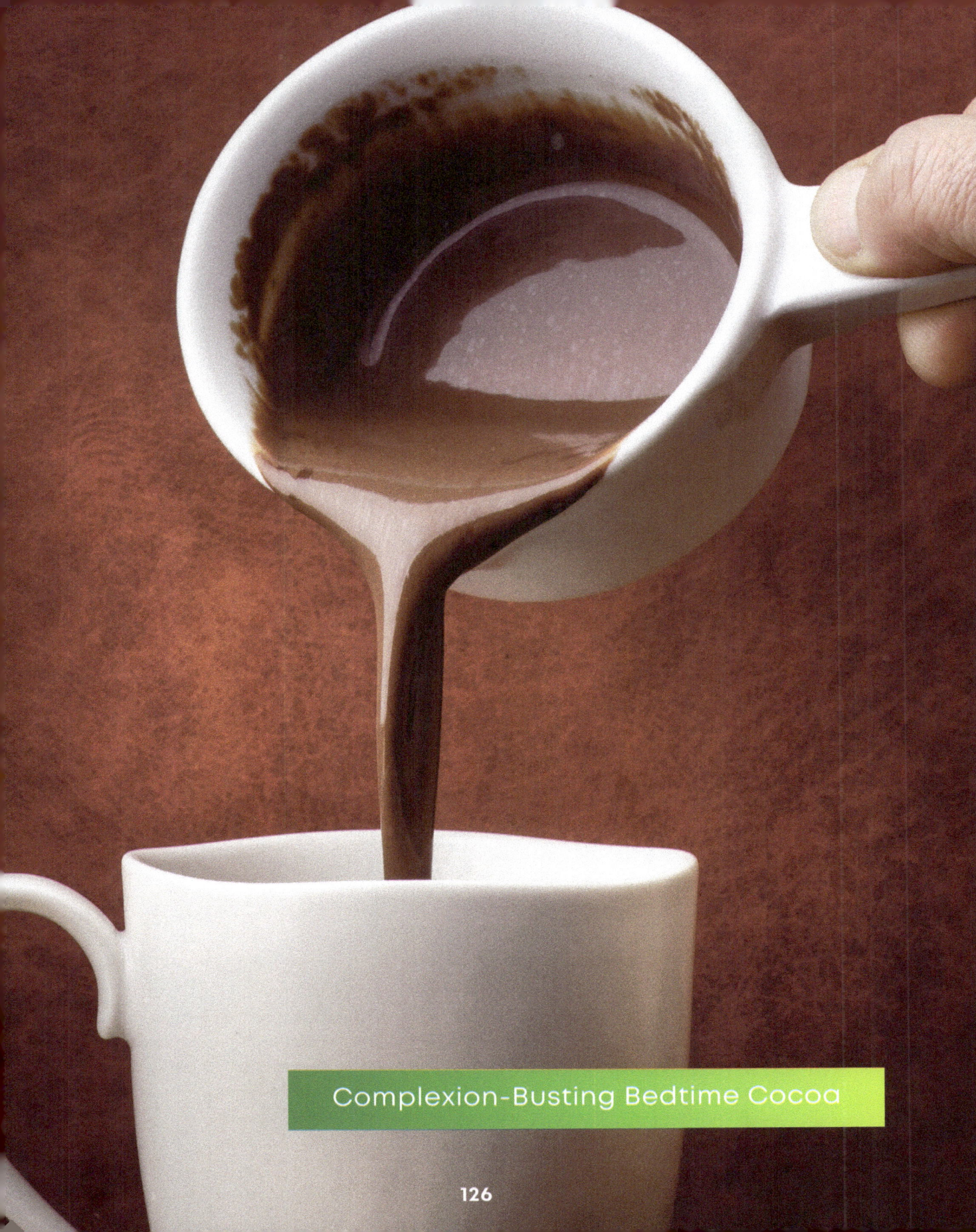

Complexion-Busting Bedtime Cocoa

Complexion-Busting Bedtime Cocoa

SERVINGS: 1

INGREDIENTS

2 tablespoons cocoa
250ml milk of your choice

METHOD

Boil the milk in a small saucepan or in the microwave.
Stir the cocoa in, sweeten if desired and enjoy.
Brilliant and comforting just before bedtime.

Cheesecake Freezer Cakes

SERVINGS: 8-12

INGREDIENTS

This makes quite a few, so keep them in the freezer until you need a treat

2 egg yolks
250g cream cheese
100ml plain yogurt
Zest and juice of one lemon
3 tablespoons sugar *or maple syrup or sweetener*
1 teaspoon vanilla extract or paste

BASE

1 packet sugar-free biscuits

METHOD

Simply blend the ingredients together until smooth.
You can make these chocolate if you like, by adding 1 tablespoon of cocoa powder.
I use a large silicone ice cube tray, but you can use any similar dishes to do small individual portions.
Place one broken biscuit into the base of each mould. Top with the smooth cream cheese filling.
Bake for about 10-12 minutes at 180C or until they have changed from glossy to matt on the top.
Allow to cool and then freeze and enjoy as little treats from time to time.

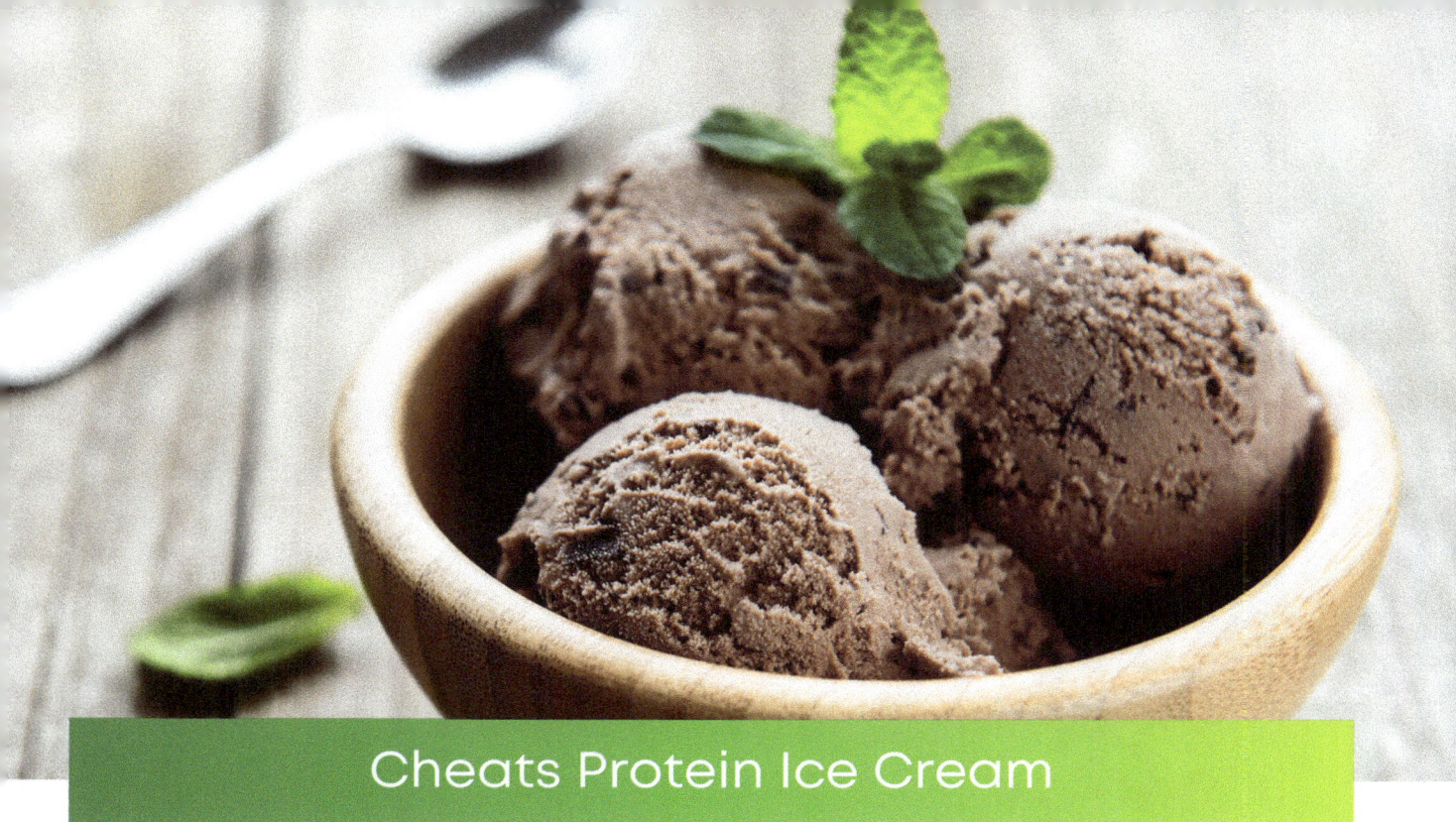

Cheats Protein Ice Cream

SERVINGS: 4-6

INGREDIENTS

1 litre milk or water
4-6 scoops protein powder
5 ml vanilla paste or extract
4 tablespoons cocoa powder OR 100 ml blended berries
OR 100 ml mango puree (you decide on the flavour...pick ONE)

METHOD

YOU DO NEED AN ICE CREAM CHURN FOR THIS RECIPE

Mix all of these ingredients together until very smooth using a strong blender.
Place the blended mixture in the freezer until nicely chilled, at least 30 minutes. Your mixture ALWAYS needs to be chilled BEFORE you ever put it into a frozen ice cream barrel for churning.
Now pour this into the frozen barrel of an ice cream churn and churn until you get a lovely soft-serve texture.
Transfer into a suitable container, and then return to the freezer until it has set.
You can freeze in smaller portions and enjoy when you need a treat.
And you can change the flavours for as many variations as you like.

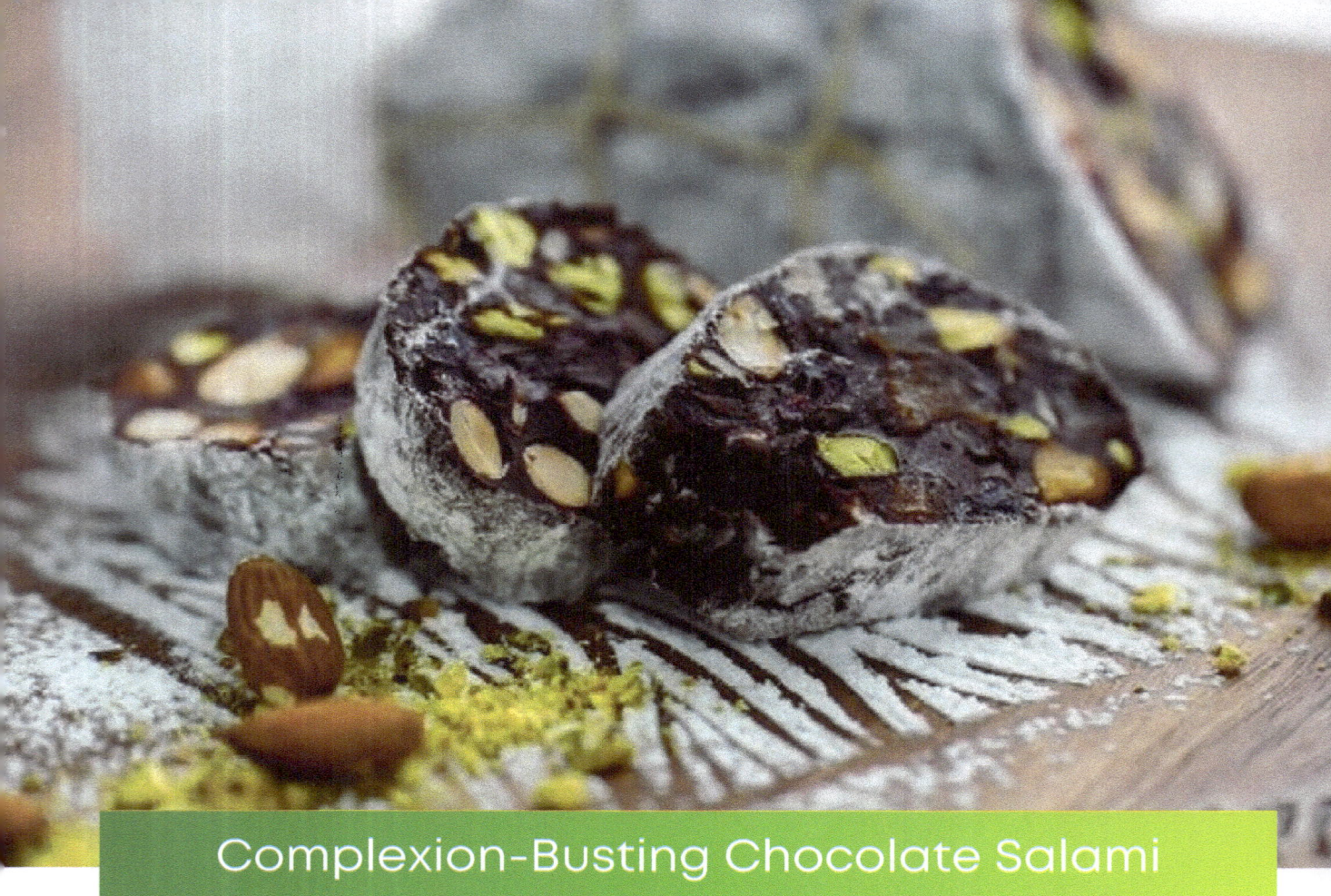

Complexion-Busting Chocolate Salami

SERVINGS: 6-8

INGREDIENTS

200g good quality chocolate (75% cocoa)
100ml coconut cream
1/2 cup toasted coconut, shredded
1/2 cup toasted cashews (unsalted)
1/2 cup pistachios or other nuts, *almonds are cheaper*
1/2 cup dates or dried fruit
1 teaspoon vanilla bean paste
Nuts, biscotti or toasted coconut, ground to a 'dust'

METHOD

Melt the chocolate in the microwave for about 1 minute until it has softened and you can stir it into a smooth paste. Add the remaining ingredients and place on a piece of parchment paper, then roll up as a 'salami', coating it in either nut dust, biscotti dust or coconut, and then chill before slicing or even rolling into 'goodie' balls… check your skin for a healthy glow soon after eating these!

NOTES

NOTES

Meet Chef Mel
THE HAPPY CHEF

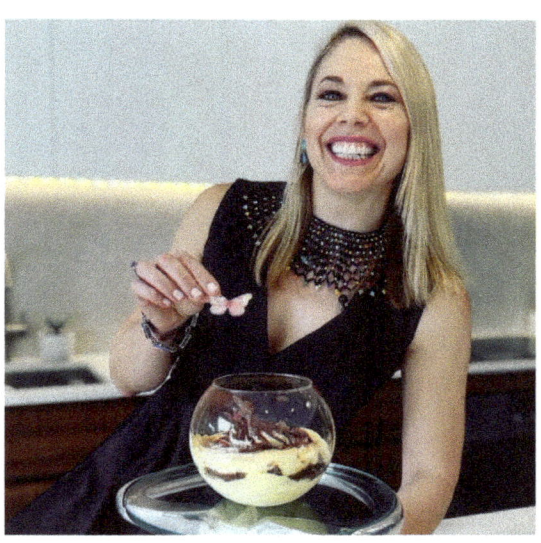

PASSIONATE FOODIE, AUTHOR, ENTREPRENEUR, COOKING SCHOOL TEACHER, ATHLETE, CULTURAL GASTRONOMER AND CHEF

With a smile that can light up a room, she has been dubbed "The Happy Chef" by her students. Chef Mel is brilliant at making everyday dishes dazzling.
Her clever approach to cooking and teaching focuses on making recipes easy to understand, with time spent on excellent presentation skills.

The enthusiastic, entertaining, award-winning, African-Australian chef and cooking school owner says that with some know-how, anyone can plate up spectacular spreads like those you would expect to see in five-star restaurants.
Her intoxicating enthusiasm, authenticity and culinary lingo will have you hungry to flex your muscles in the kitchen.

She promises that this book will teach you some seriously cheffy skills so that you will be so much more confident and happy in your kitchen.

She can't wait to help you become the foodie you have always wanted to be!

Get ready to make delicious discoveries!

www.ingramcontent.com/pod-product-compliance
Lightning Source LLC
Chambersburg PA
CBHW061136010526
44107CB00068B/2966